POCKET GUIDE TO FITNESS

All You Need to Know to Start Working Out Effectively

By Louiza Patsis, M. S.

Bloomington, IN

authorHOUSE®

Milton Keynes, UK

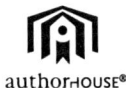

AuthorHouse™
1663 Liberty Drive, Suite 200
Bloomington, IN 47403
www.authorhouse.com
Phone: 1-800-839-8640

AuthorHouse™ UK Ltd.
500 Avebury Boulevard
Central Milton Keynes, MK9 2BE
www.authorhouse.co.uk
Phone: 08001974150

First published by AuthorHouse 3/5/2007

ISBN: 978-1-4259-5675-2 (sc)

*Printed in the United States of America
Bloomington, Indiana*

This book is printed on acid-free paper.

This book is dedicated to my late great father Dionysios Sotiris Patsis, a man of love, integrity, talent and sense of humor.

Contents

Introduction

I have been working out for years. It is something that I love to do. I remember that at 18 years old, although I looked great and had no problem getting a date, I would huff and puff after jogging around one block, or I would get on the stationary bicycle at my university dormitory gym for about 10 minutes and sweat. Since I started to go to the gym regularly, my endurance, strength and flexibility have greatly improved. Going to the gym is a place to be by myself, do something by myself and connect my spiritual, mental and physical sides of my being into a multi-dimensional whole. It has allowed me to take part in hobbies such as hiking, skiing and jogging, including long-distance runs. My energy level has increased. I can often work, study and go out with little sleep for days.

I am at a point that I can generally regulate the amount of muscle and fat in my body. I can control my weight without expensive programs or diet fads. And I feel good about myself at any weight.

I would like to share some of what I have learned with you. I kept a blog of fitness from October 2005. This book is derived from the blog.

Louiza Patsis, M.S.

Disclaimer:

Part I

Spiritual and Mental Aspects of Working Out

A. Your Spirit and Your Work Out: Be Non-Attached

Many people think that working out only is a physical activity. Well, it is also spiritual and mental. Let's focus on the spiritual now. What will give you that extra push to work out if you are in pain? What will keep you committed to your work out? It is your spirit — you will to increase the level of your fitness, the fight in you to keep going when it gets touch, the belief in yourself that you can reach your goals, the love for yourself when you fail a goal, and the capacity to recommit. All of that extends from your spirit.

Have you ever watched athletes? They are talented, of course, or they would not get where they are and they would not get paid millions of dollars. But what keeps them going when they are tired? What keeps them going when they are losing the game and all eyes are on them? What makes them get up when they lose and be able to play another game? What keeps them going is their spirit. In fact, when you work out, you are working out your spirit, character, brain and personality as much as you are working out your body. You are exercising the love and commitment to yourself, your integrity in health, your commitment power, and your strength.

Working out does not have to be about work. It can be about commitment to your health and your goals, not an attachment that things like your body and work outs, and goal attainment have to look a certain way. When you are attached, you often suffer. Working out is not fun. You don't like yourself if you don't meet your goals. As you work out, you may be able to get to the point where you BE working out. It is a part of you—not a task. It is the air you breathe. Strive for that, but do not be attached! Have fun at your work out.

B. Hitting the Wall During the Marathon or Anywhere Else

If you have run for a long distance, you know that after a period of time, you hit a "wall". The time you hit this may be later the more you practice. The wall can be caused by fatigue or by different muscles each time. Often when you run, it is caused by your feet! I find that no matter what sneakers you buy, they will hurt!

As I emphasize often, work outs are spiritual and mental as well as physical. When I have run marathons, I often find myself thinking about people and things that affect me for miles! It's great that I can catch myself doing this and get it out of my mind. It is also wonderful to be with the people and energy of New York City. But I am telling you: learning to master your spirit and mind can have you master your body.

If you find yourself hitting a wall at a long-distance run, or in an emotional state, relationship or at work, breathe, identify your feelings, be with them and be present to or create a commitment that is larger than the feelings and wall. At the same time, enjoy the moment.

Challenge yourself to surpass the wall. You can start with increments. Tell yourself you will cross a certain landmark, and in how much time. Connect with Nature and people around you.

You will find that the wall disappears, or at least gets smaller! Practice.

C. Failure

Failure can be good. We all fail, often many times, before we accomplish what we set out to do. Each time we fail, we grow in the following ways: 1. Who we are regarding failure gives us growth; 2. We see what our triggers of failure from the past are; 3. We evolve in our relationship to failure; 4. We see what was missing and put it in to be more effective next time; and 5. We learn from our experience, grow and mature as human beings.

By failing we get to see if we are really committed to our goals and not attached. If we are attached, we get to see how we self-sabotage our commitment. What self-sabotaging conversations do we have? These can include:

I will never be good enough.

It is too good to be true.

I do not have the time.

I do not know how.

I cannot do it.

D. Hard Work

Do you know how sometimes you do not want to take the first step? You may not want to start a conversation with someone and talk about something that you both have been avoiding. You may not want to start that term paper. You may not want to start your workout. But the first step is the most important step.

You may find that all of that hard work that you are avoiding is really just in your mind. Look back on your life to when you were happy. Happiness is generated from the inside, but that will be in another. You may find that you were happy relaxing at the beach or on the patio with a lemonade, or talking with a friend on a lazy afternoon. You may also find that you were happy when you "worked hard". Many people get a high from sweating and doing the work — doing what needs to be done to get a promotion, finish that report, build some muscle.

Everything is yin/yang. Intending results and being a big, welcoming receptor for results is more of the yin quality of human beings and the Universe. The reverse of that is action — going out and creating and doing what it takes to get what you want. Think of a great football player scoring a touchdown. First he catches the ball while other football players are trying to block him or hit him. Then he maneuvers his way against all the obstacles on the field to make that touchdown. All the while, he stays mindful and present. From the beginning, he intended and was committed to making a great play and scoring, or at least contributing to his team winning. The flip side of that was the action, the challenge with himself, and the competitive drive. Spirit, mind and action are involved in making your goals happen.

Recently, I resisted starting to work on one of the several papers that I have to complete for the end of this semester in my Ph.D. program in information science. It took months to get the books I needed, and hours to read them and make notes for the paper. Then I had to organize my major points, write, edit and type! Once I took the first step, the rest was a good flow of "hard work" I actually enjoyed snuggling up in my bed and creating that paper.

The same can be true for working out. Take that first step. Start to work. You may find you love the "hard work" and sweat, until it is not hard work anymore and becomes your self-expression! Be happy and be your "work" moment to moment!

E. Choose Your Body!

Choosing where you are is important. You can be in traffic, and whine, curse and complain. Doing so to an extent is not "bad". After all, complaining does several things: it gives us an access to who we are, our needs, and wants; it offers us an opportunity for some intimacy and sharing with close ones; and it gives us an opportunity to see things that we are not fond of in life, and a chance to transform them or go get what we want!

At the same time, we can choose where we are and trust the Universe that we are exactly where we need to be. This includes our bodies. This comes down to loving yourself. After all, many people do not have their health, and doing something as simple as breathing or walking is difficult. Our bodies are miracles. Love your body. There is only one you in the Universe. Love yourself! You are beautiful! And if someone else says that you are not, so what? Think so! And if you don't think so – think so! You will end up believing it!

Unless you love and accept your body before taking on working out, one of the following will happen: You struggle in and hate the process of losing weight; you try and try again, and your weight keeps yo-yoing; you never lose weight; or you lose weight, keep the weight off, yet are never truly free and happy.

After you accept your body, whatever shape you are in, you get to choose how you want to look. Do not forget that, before starting an exercise program, you must get a medical check-up. This includes if you have had one at any time before six months. Health is most important. If you have a bad back or knee and the physician, chiropractor, or physical therapist tell you not to do certain exercises, listen to them. You get to set the goals for yourself. You do not have to look like anyone you know or anyone in a magazine.

F. Perfection Context and Being Straight with Yourself

This is related to the section called "Choose Your Body". Do you ever think that everything you do, whether it is raising your children, cleaning your home, looking good, losing weight or your body is never good enough? Do you think you will never get the body you want?

There is a difference between striving for perfection, thinking you will attain it after you take several steps or thinking you will never attain it, and being straight with yourself in terms of something you need to put into action to up the level of what you are doing. I think of myself as perfect from the spiritually, mentally, emotionally and physically. I rejoice in who I am and always did since I was a child. I can lose or gain weight, be tired, laugh or yell, and at the core of my being, the context of what I do, that is what I believe.

We are marvelous creatures. No two of us are alike, even identical twins. We came out of one sperm meeting an egg of a particular month, and we are here! Our bodies are an amazingly complex and coordinated system. Have you ever thought how lucky you are to be here and to be healthy, or to have the level of health that you have?

Why not think of yourself as perfect? I do not mean to have severe acne and think you will make it to the cover of a dermatology magazine. I do not mean to not work out for months and notice you are huffing and puffing up the stairs and not go to the physician. I do not mean to not get to the source of your losing your temper. I do not mean to like how your hair looks a certain style and not go to the hairdresser. I do not mean to not be straight with yourself when you are being lazy, or to not think that there is something you can put in like an ingredient to a recipe that can up the level of what you are doing, if that is your commitment.

I mean to really feel and get that you are special and perfect. It may not be explainable in words.

Do you get it?

G. Success = Getting Up Over and Over Again

Working out ultimately is not about looking good. It is about health and it is about looking good. Ultimately it is a way of being. It is growth. It is connected in several dimensions to mentality and spirituality. One thing you get about working out is to stay committed to your goals, forgive yourself when you do not meet them, and get back up over and over again. If you do not do this, you are quitting, and missing one of the many lessons that working out gives to you. Even if you work out alone, you grow and learn from working out. You apply the lessons to life, family, work, fun and everything!

This is a valuable lesson that you do not want to miss. Whether you do not reach your fitness goals or weight goals, or you miss a day, or you do not get an exercise right, or you feel pain after an exercise, or whatever else, you will learn, as long as you are present and aware, to get back up over and over again.

Success is defined by culture and media. It often means for people to look good, have great relationships, have money and have things. None of these aspects of success are inherently bad. YOU get to define success for yourself. And an important element of that is to forgive and love yourself, and to get back up over and over again.

H. Get to Know Yourself

Working out is not just about health, looking good and getting bigger and stronger. Its benefits include mental and the spiritual elements.

When you work out in one hour, one day, one week, one year, or years, through the same or different routines, outdoor sports, aerobics classes, free weights or anything else, you get to know yourself. That is one of the huge benefits of working out.

What do I mean by getting to know yourself? Have you ever overcome a big obstacle? Have you overcome heartbreak, relatives that are a way that does not work for you, a boss who acts like a jerk, tough courses in school, an illness or any other situation? Well, that is like sticking with your workout, finishing a Marathon, going when you see no results yet.

Like peeling the layers of an onion, with you being the onion, you get to see who you are, what you are made of, what makes you tick, and what you can do. And that is priceless.

I. Acknowledge Yourself

You must acknowledge yourself when you go to the gym. If you fail to meet a weight loss goal by a set time, acknowledge yourself for trying, getting to the gym and being a person who plays and fights. If you are in a game, race or long-distance run, acknowledge yourself.

If you finish a workout and feel pain, acknowledge and love yourself. If you miss some days at the gym, forgive yourself for even playing the fitness game and noticing you were out of integrity.

You are healthy enough to move. Even if you are sick, you love, you think, and you move. You are amazing. You are "lucky". You are unique and the only one of you in the world. You are taking on your health. You are you. You are the "luckiest" person on Earth.

You are beautiful. You are fun. You mean business. You play to win but are always a winner! You are the best. You are real. You get to the bottom of things and play. Acknowledge yourself.

J. Be Grateful

Did you ever notice how beautiful birds are when they sit on a winter tree branch and munch on a little berry? Did you notice how new rain and snow often are even if you have seen them before hundreds of times? Did you notice how your eyes, nose, toes and other body parts are unique and your own? You would notice them anytime and anywhere!

Do you know how even the pain after some workouts feels good? Does it feel great for you to know you did what you said that you would do in terms of working out? Doesn't it feel good to breathe, be alive and be healthy? Isn't the spring breeze or winter wind on your face an expression of love in the Universe?

It is all good. Be grateful.

K. Dance! Be in the Moment!

I went dancing for the first time in weeks last night. I went to the Copa Cabana after office work dressed in sexy but not-too-sexy clothes and long boots. And I danced, and danced, and danced. I was not too attracted to my partner, but I danced. I could have easily said that I wanted to go home and sleep but I danced. I thought that I wanted to go home, but I stayed and danced.

I connected to myself. I was in the moment. I felt past dates and pains and regrets. But I danced. I expressed who I am. I felt my strength, used it and shared it with the world. I expressed my sexuality. When my partner paused to wipe off his sweat, I danced.

At times like this, there is the present moment. Who cares if you blew your workout yesterday? Who cares if you have a report due at work today? You are here now lifting that free weight. You are great, strong, committed, and present. Dance! Be true to who you are! Be true to your word! Get in the game of your life. Get into your work out. Be it. Perform. Breathe. You are done. Congratulate yourself.

Dancing is wonderful for spirit, mind, emotions and body. You express yourself, gain in confidence, and cardiovascular fitness and muscular strength. You connect with yourself and with other people if you choose. You connect with and show your full range of emotions that are part of being human, and that we often hide (sometimes thankfully) in everyday life. It is also a great flexibility exercise.

Your muscles have memory. A ballerina can do things that a football player will find hard to do and a football player will do things that a ballerina will find hard to do. Each time you use a muscle in a different way and angle, you hit different muscle fibers and that muscle will grow and be stronger. Dancing at different rhythms and tempos can be a great form of interval training. You can go slow and then quickly. You can move and stretch muscles, increasing the level of muscle flexibility and strength.

You can monitor your level of expertise in a dance. This will increase your connection to yourself spiritually, mentally, emotionally and physically. You will gain in knowing the distinctions of confidence, commitment, discipline, beauty, self-expression, creativity and more.

You can do all of this while you have fun, and even enjoy it with a partner or with a group of people! And of course you have the music to go along with it!

Working out is the best hobby. It prepares you for times like this, to dance!

You never know what can happen!

L. Express Yourself!

What is your self-expression? Millions of people are not expressing themselves in their work. You can see it in their faces in the subway in New York City. They do not look inspired. When some people wear a uniform, they do not feel like they are expressing themselves. I remember that I had to wear a uniform in Catholic high school where I had to wear a uniform. We had to wear collars. So I tore off an old white shirt and put its collar under a tank top. I had several detentions for uniforms my freshman year. The Dean of Women finally forgot about it and let me on my way. I was a good student.

What is your expression for your body? It need not be a "cookie cutter" body like that of aerobics instructors. By "cookie cutter" I mean a body that looks like many other bodies. It seems like people are striving for that. One of the earliest sections was about how no two people have the same genetics or bodies. One person has a color eyes that no one has seen, and another person has a particular shape of biceps that no one has seen. One person may have a big bottom. Several celebrities have made money off their distinct features. Love what is your own and what you cannot change, except perhaps by drastic measures. Then choose what you want and can change.

What is your true self-expression? Is it being a big bodybuilder? Is it being a welterweight boxer? Is it being slim with few muscles? Is it being voluptuous? First get your annual medical check-ups, connect with yourself to monitor how you feel and perform, and then choose what workout you want for the body you want. And love yourself!

M. Learn to Listen to Your Body!

It is important to get to know your body through working out to know if pain you may feel is real pain or just an excuse. If it is real pain, you should stop working out or rest. See a physician or physical therapist if the pain is excruciating or preventing you from doing what you want to do. Spirituality, meditating, martial arts and more can have you learning to know yourself more. Working out is key. Just as we often do not listen to ourselves or to other people "cleanly", we do the same with our bodies. For instance, if your mother tells you to wear a coat, you may think she is being a nagging old woman. She barely has a chance to tell you that she heard something informative on the weather channel.

People may listen to their bodies like their bodies do not know what they are telling them or they may ignore their bodies. Through working out, you will learn to listen to when you are really hungry, when you need to eat what, when you are really in pain and when you need to work out what.

For instance, a person who has muscle and is not sleeping much, is undergoing stress, or is using lots of glucose for their brain may be able or even need to eat something sugary while studying at night. This energy may be burned. I have skipped a meal or two while studying for my Ph.D. courses. At least twice I was nauseous because acid in my stomach "wanted" something to digest. At other times I became drowsy while driving home. Many times while studying and staying up late while maintaining my workout schedule of about every other day, at least 65 minutes working out at the gym, I can eat late at night, including sugary foods, and I end up losing weight!

Learn to listen to yourself. Months ago I saw that I was dreading doing squats, which I usually did on Mondays. I know that I will make sure I work out through most pain and will not let myself get lazy. But this was a real dread that my physical intuition was telling me. I found from a physical therapist and a Rolfing person that I have slight arthritis in my knees, especially right one which I suspected for years. I have not been doing squats for some months now. If I see that my legs are losing muscle or strength, I will make sure that I up my leg exercises or reinstate squats with less weight and more repetitions.

You will understand this fully by experience. Learn to listen to your body.

N. Pain

Lots of people dread pain. So what do they do? They avoid it? Lots of these same people are the ones that sign up for a gym membership only to go a few times before going back to relaxing on the couch. If someone starts working out for the first time ever or in years, the old adage "No pain, no gain" may be true. And if you want to lose weight, you most often have to sweat. So that means that doing the stationary bicycle on Level Zero for 20 minutes a day may do close to nothing for healthy, fit individuals.

If you want muscle gain in strength and size, you often have to take your muscle beyond the work it usually does. Muscle fibers may tear and grow back, stronger and larger. You may feel pain that day or the next.

One of the most invaluable things about working out is that you get to know your body and yourself. You get to know what is bogus pain and what is real pain. For instance, if your toe or your stomach hurts a little, if you have a slight back pain or if you are a little drowsy and have a slight headache, that can be an excuse not to work out. There are times that I had pneumonia, a severe cold, little sleep, and major back pain, and I worked out. Now I don't suggest you do the same thing. I have been working out for years. But do not fool yourself into making excuses for yourself.

Rest is very important. If you have true pain or really need rest, skip a day at the gym. The pain can be good news: it can show you that you really need to see a physician or a chiropractor, rest, sleep or do something to de-stress. Learn to listen to yourself. And you bet you will, the more you work out!

O. Payoff

We all have payoffs in doing or in not doing something. Often the payoff for putting something off is to have the opportunity to whine about it and to have others make us feel better. Another way in which a payoff can be used is that we want what we want now. I have the same characteristic. My father told me to be humble and to be patient. I am still working on those virtues.

We often want to see results soon. For instance, we may want to see that "cut" in our triceps when we look backward into the mirror. We can work out those triceps each day, but chances are that they will fatigue and that we will not want to work them out for months. I believe that the pendulum with everything swings back the other way when there is no balance.

We can learn yet something else by working out: patience. We can work out those triceps and rest them a day or even two in between. Then we can wait months to see those "cuts" in the back of the arms. And you know what, all that work and time will be worth it! And we will have greater confidence ahead!

P. Setting Goals: Don't Stop!

Did you ever think that you cannot reach the goal of, let's say, losing that final five pounds, giving up smoking, giving up sugar, or losing a clothing size?

I have written a lot about accepting and loving yourself. That does not mean not reaching for your goals! Now if you did not meet a goal, acknowledge yourself, and set another goal! That's right! Do not give up!

It may be true that you had to work extra late for work and could not find time for the gym. It can be valid, or it can be an excuse. After some months of working out, you should know the difference, just like you can know the difference between real and "excuse" pain. For instance, if you had to work a lot, perhaps you could have eaten less fats or found time in the morning for a short run.

You have to love yourself and be committed, but with no action, often there are no results! So do what the Nike commercial says: Just do it! Get up and recommit!

Often for Lent, I give something up. That can be something I love or am used to, like chocolate or red meat. (I do not eat a lot of red meat, but usually do not exclude it entirely.) After a day or two, it gets to be easy. The same can be said for a new diet, like a low-carbohydrate diet. For the first few days, you probably will be irritated and drowsy and go to sleep at around 7:30 pm. But after a few days on the diet, you will get used to it and love it!

Often what blocks our goals is psychological. Get to the source of it by getting to know yourself, listening to your intuition and talking to a friend or a professional.

Either way, forgive yourself for not reaching a goal, create another one, and seriously go after it with fun!

Q. Sports

Individual and group sports are great. They can be a wonderful way to work out and a way to get off a plateau. I used to think that sports and watching sports were silly, until I was about 22 years old and I started to go to a gym regularly! I also at one point thought that eating most vegetables was yucky or that acting was for idiots that were not smart. I turned around some time in my early twenties. That shows you to never say "never".

It can be magical and miraculous to see accomplished athletes alone or in teams playing sports. These people are clear, focused powerhouses. Besides being entertainment, excellence in sports is something inspiring to strive for and is a metaphor for health, relationships and business.

Some individual sports are hiking, dancing, handball, skiing and roller blading. Some team sports are baseball, volleyball, football and tennis. Some sports can be done alone or in groups — skating, racket sports against a wall or with partners(s), hiking and more.

The more in shape you are, the better and longer you can engage in sports. It is a wonderful experience to feel muscles that you never felt before and to see that you can do something that you could not do the past year. Individual and group sports will increase your confidence, intellect, instincts, endurance, flexibility, coordination and strength. Team sports will give you distinctions in love, partnership and appreciation for yourself and other people.

While engaging in sports, as when you work out, you will connect your spiritual, mental, emotional and physical parts. You will be your word in what goals you set for yourself, learn to fail and succeed, commit, and have fun! You can meet people too!

R. Educate Yourself!

There is so much power in knowledge. And there is even more power in knowledge and experience and knowing yourself. I was at a recent gathering of beauty queens and their consultants. I was so happy to hear these young women talking about inner beauty, eating what they want in moderation according to what they need and not wearing a lot of makeup.

Much of health, fitness and beauty is about loving and standing for yourself. One way to do this is to spend the time to go to the library, search the Internet or ask an expert like a physician, dietician, yoga teacher and personal trainer about fitness. There is so much power in knowing what is happening inside your body when you eat or exercise, in knowing about different exercises, and in knowing your body and how it works with food and exercise.

As with working out, there may be a hesitance or phobia of science. Remember, the only way to know how anything is going to be and if you will like it is to take the step and do it! You may find out that you love learning, researching and working out! They are your power! And they are fun!

Part II

Fitness Facts

Miscellaneous Fitness Tips
to Get You Going

A. Your Personal Trainer and You

Do you need a personal trainer? Well, this depends on your fitness level and knowledge. If you are a novice going to the gym, or pursuing a new sport, it is an excellent idea to get a personal trainer or coach. A good personal trainer will make sure that you have an okay from a physician to work out. Then they will ask you what you want to do: tone up, have arms that are more cut, trim your waist, run a marathon, hike, be more flexible, become a size four or whatever YOU want. The personal trainer or coach can be there to see the greatness in a person even if the person does not see it on her or his own. Her or his job is to show you their knowledge, monitor your posture and results, see what works for you and empower you in your motivation. It is your job to be motivated, to say how you feel, to get to know your body, to monitor your own results as well, and to be disciplined in being on time and following your routine and diet (if assigned a special one). It is also your job to get to know the cardiovascular and weight routines and equipment, and to get to know what muscle does what, how to stretch and rest your muscles, and how a fitness program works. That way, when the time comes, you can fly from the nest. In a year or less, it is usually best for a client to be on their own and follow the program and even add to it or modify it by themselves. This will give the client a sense of independence. If you have a new fitness goal, then go ahead and hire or take on another personal trainer or coach for a while. Otherwise, once you get to know the tricks, be on your own. You can do it!

B. Perhaps the Best Abdominal Exercise

Many people have trouble with their abdominal muscles. This includes women that have just had a baby. It also includes men that have a "beer belly", if you will. The first thing to do if you have excess fat on your midsection is to do cardiovascular work to sweat and burn the calories.

This is something that now all people understand: If you have a lot of muscle tissue in your abdominal wall, it will not show if you have a layer of fat that will not let it show. If a bodybuilder, for instance, competes in a bodybuilding contest, she or he will trim down the days before the event. More muscles will show. Another thing that some people do not understand is that women, even fit women, tend to have more fat or a thicker layer of fat than men. Even if the women have a good set of abdominal muscles, they will not show a six-pack unless they trim down more, often losing fat from their face, chest, and other areas from which they do not want to lose fat.

Abdominal muscles are often secondary muscles in many moves — such as lying down and lifting your legs up and down. Sit-ups and other exercises can be used to target abdominal muscles as primary movers. Here is an exercise in which abdominal muscles are both primary and secondary movers and is one of the best abdominal exercises out there. It is an advanced exercise. Do not do this exercise without the approval of your physician.

To stretch, stand up and reach up for a few seconds at least three separate times. Sit sideways on a chair, with its back to your right or left. Place your gluteus maximus on the edge of the chair. Place your hands behind your head. Lift your shoulders and legs up at the same time. Support your head with your hands and keep your elbows out parallel to your ribcage as much as possible. Do four sets of ten abdominal sit-ups this way. Increase the amount of repetitions every four weeks by five repetitions per set, if you are an intermediate exerciser in terms of your abdominal muscles. Or increase the repetitions as you see fit for the exercise to give you a burn and to be possible to do!

Here is an advanced isometric movement: During one of the repetitions per set, hold the position with your shoulders and knees as close together as possible for about five seconds. This varies the workout. This movement and isometric movements are tough. Isometric movements should only be done for seconds at a time and once in a while and only by intermediate or advanced exercisers. To stretch, stand up and reach up for a few seconds at least three separate times.

This is a tough exercise! When you are done, pat yourself on the back!

C. Plateaus Are Not Only in Arizona

Have you ever started to eat ravenously? Then you get stuffed halfway through the meal and start feeling full, heavy, or even sick. But you go on. Then the high you first felt goes away and you are just flat. You are happy to be eating so the food does not go to waste. But there is no more fun. Have you ever felt a relationship get stale after awhile? Either the sex is no fun or the conversation reveals nothing new about the other person or nothing exhilarating and inspiring.

Something similar can happen when you work out. If you do the same routine for over three months, six months, or especially one year, you may see that your body — endurance, muscle growth and vitality — does not respond as it first did. And you may end up feeling bored. Some people—those that lack motivation and drive, or those that simply are not turned on about the workout and need to be to keep going — will decrease the amount of days working out or stop working out altogether!

Everyone's medical health, fitness, body and goals differ. For a healthy person approved to work out by their physician, who wants to tone up and lose excess fat, workout routines should be changed every three or four weeks, then more dramatically every three to four months, and then even more each year. That does not mean that you have to change something that works for you, such as running a certain amount of hours on the treadmill every week. It could mean small, subtle changes like varying the incline on the treadmill, incorporating arm movements, or changing the leg weight exercises you do that day. It could mean running outside for a periods of some weeks or months. Changing your workout routine could be varying the abdominal exercises you do or using a Swiss ball with abdominal exercises for some weeks or months.

At first you may need to work with a personal trainer to design your workout for some weeks, months or a year. Now if you are injured or really feel you want to maintain where you are in fitness, a plateau is not a definite no-no. A primary idea in working out is to really get to know and feel your body, and to be able to design your own workouts.

Take a trip to Arizona to see those mesmerizing plateaus. But don't have them in your workouts!

D. Variations

Variations of exercises are very important. Each time you vary any exercise, from a biceps curl to a squat, you get off a little plateau and work out new muscle fibers of muscle fibers in a new angle. I will not get into the biomechanics of this in this pocket guide. You can consult a textbook. You can also try it for yourself and see how it feels.

Here are three examples:

1. Biceps curls: Do some while curving your wrists outward. See what new parts of your biceps muscles are targeted. Do not forget to stretch before and after. This can be done by putting your arm shoulder level or one inch higher with your thumb against the wall and moving your body away from your arm. Hold for at least three seconds.

2. Push-ups using medicine ball: Hold medicine balls while you do push-ups. Some medicine balls come with handles. It is especially challenging to perform this exercise without handles. Try it both ways if you can. This makes the exercise more difficult since you have to work on stabilizing the balls. Now try just one ball at the time. This varies the pectoral and oblique muscle fibers used. Don't forget to stretch before and after: hold your arms behind your chest and grasp your hands together. Stick your chest out. Hold for at least three seconds.

3. Leg extensions: This is for your quadriceps. Try pointing your toes in or out and doing the repetitions. This varies quadriceps muscle fibers used. Don't forget to stretch before and after: hold each leg ankle behind you one at a time. Hold for at least ten seconds for each leg.

E. Interval Training

Interval training is an amazing way to increase your cardiovascular health, get off a plateau and increase performance in day-to-day life or in a sport. It is sometimes called Guerilla Cardio or, by the Swedes, the Fartlek technique. It is to be used by intermediate or advanced exercisers, and done for the first few times after the permission of a physician and the overseeing of a personal trainer. An interval session involves a warm-up period, several short, maximum-intensity efforts separated by moderate recovery intervals, and a cool down period. At the beginning, the total time can be just five minutes and one can work themselves up to 40 minutes. Besides the above health benefits, it is proven to be more effective at burning calories compared to long duration, low intensity workouts.

Interval training is a way to improve your aerobic capacity, which is the ability of the body to remove oxygen from the air and transfer it through the lungs and blood to the working muscles. You will raise your anaerobic threshold, the point at which the body can no longer meet its demand for oxygen. Thus, you will be able to keep utilizing oxygen in aerobic respiration, which burns fat! And you will be able to work out harder and longer.

You can use many movements in interval training and incorporate it creatively into a cardiovascular or weight workout. You can walk or run slowly for some minutes, and then quickly, alternating speeds. The fast walk or sprint run can last about a minute. You can use climbing and descending stairs slowly and quickly, or use this quickly in between ten-minute cardiovascular session. You can incorporate walking, running and climbing stairs. Spin classes often use interval training by varying speed and incline.

Go past your comfort zone. But, as with everything else in working out, listen to your body. If real injury can occur, cool down or stop. You will see that each time, or every few times, that you do interval training, you will get better at it. You can use a heart rate monitor to make sure that you stay in your target heart rate zone.

To find out more about the science of interval training, look it up at www.pubmed.gov.

F. Climb the Stairs!

Even if you are a beginner, it is easy to incorporate interval training into your exercise routine. Incorporating it is easy, of course, but actually doing it may be tough. Start off slowly. Ask a physician's permission first, as when you go for your annual physical check-up. Here are some ways to incorporate interval training in your exercise routines:

For cardiovascular training:
>   You can alter the speed and – or incline on a treadmill for a minute or for two minutes. You can alter the speed and resistance on a stationary bicycle for a minute or for two minutes. You can alter the

resistance on a stairmaster for a minute or for two minutes.

For weight training:

In between sets, you can do one of the following activities. Choose one per day or week.

Activity One:

Jog in place. Do this for a minute or two minutes between sets.

Activity Two:

Run up and down the stairs. Do this for a minute or two minutes between sets.

Activity Three:

Jump rope. Do this for a minute or two minutes between sets.

Activity Four:

Put on boxing gloves. Hit a punching bag. Do this for a minute or two minutes between sets.

G. Plyometrics: A Great Way to Increase Power and to De-Plateau

Plyometrics are any exercise where the muscle is contracted eccentrically, and then is immediately, contracted concentrically. The muscle is stretched (i.e., loaded) before it is contracted. An example of this is doing lunges or squats quickly one after the other, with the motion of straightening up (not fully by straightening the knees) being almost a jump. Plyometrics increase power. Power is strength or work times speed, or how much you can lift or how much energy you expend in what period of time. The faster this is, the more power you have. Power is important if you want to take off at a quick speed or if you want to quickly lift a falling piece of furniture before it gets your foot!

Plyometrics places increased stretch loads on the working muscles. As the muscles become more tolerant to the increase loads, the stretch-shortening cycle becomes more efficient and power increases. You should warm up with stretching or jogging or jumping rope before plyometrics.

Sprints are plyometrics since the action going down loads the hamstring muscles. Doing push-ups with claps in between main movements and jumping (especially is the low movement is very low) are other plyometrics exercises. Catching a medicine ball thrown quickly and throwing it back quickly is also a plyometrics exercise. The further back and then forward your arms go, the more advanced is the movement, as long as you do not throw yourself off balance or use momentum instead of strength. Remember to use smooth, steady motions instead of jerky ones.

Plyometrics exercises are great if you want to do something different and get off that plateau. These exercises should be done by intermediate and advanced fitness people.

H. Women, Fitness and Fat

Women tend to have more fat than men. First of all, they have their chest and hips. If you are like me, you tend to think this is how it ought to be, and that a woman does not have to be straight or pencil-thin to be healthy. Women probably have developed an extra layer of fat than men to protect a growing fetus.

Actually, one cannot tell by looking at someone if they are fit. Think of all of those athletes that have had heart problems at what you think is their utmost shape. One has to get a medical examination and perhaps take radiological tests to really know how healthy they are. They can also look at family history, strength, endurance, flexibility and more.

If a woman (or man) is healthy and fit at a certain weight and she goes from say, 120 pounds to 140 pounds, while she still works out, it does not necessarily mean she is now not as fit. First of all, muscle weighs more than fat. So it can just mean that they gained muscle! An extra inch of fat here and there does not mean that a person is out of shape or obese.

Fat is a nutrient, just like carbohydrates and protein. At nine calories per gram, it supplies more calories per gram than the other two proteins. Fat is essential for the body. It provides the "essential" fatty acids. These are not made by the body and must be obtained from food. Linoleic acid is the most important essential fatty acid. Among other things, it assists in the growth and development of infants. From fatty acids are made the molecules that are essential in the control of blood pressure, blood clotting, inflammation, and other body functions. Fat stores vitamins A, D, E and K. Fat maintains healthy skin and hair. It insulates nerve cells and helps in proper nerve functioning. It surrounds and cushions our organs, protecting them from damage. It serves as the storage substance for the body's extra calories. It insulates us against cold and against falls. (I suggest forcing yourself to sit if you are about to fall, if you have some cushioning!) Fat is the energy source your body turns to after carbohydrate calories are used, which is after about 20 minutes of exercise.

There appears to be a phobia of fat in the world. Often, what we resist persists. Each person has to find a range of body fat percent that suits them, in which they are healthy and fit, and feel great. This does not mean to be pencil thin. For some people, it is genetic to be very thin and they are healthy and look great that way as well. I believe that, for most people, being very thin is not necessarily healthy. This does not mean to eat junk food all day and marry the couch. The middle road is usually the best.

Women usually bear the brunt of skinny fads. Perhaps you can send me comments on if you think that being pencil-thin is healthy or appealing.

For now, educate yourselves on health and on your bodies. Do not be lazy, but do not be a diet or exercise fanatic either!

Some material from this section was obtained from the National Institutes of Health.

http://www.nlm.nih.gov/medlineplus/ency/
    article/002468.htm.

Accessed November 9, 2005

I. How Many Calories Should You Burn Per Day?

The amount of calories that you need per day to be healthy varies by: if you are female or male; if you are a pregnant female; your health; your diet; your age; the amount of muscle that you have; and your level of activity. Pregnant women, sick people, young and older people, and people with a high level or activity or stress need more calories than average. Men need more calories than women. This is important since the basic way to lose weight is to take in more calories and to burn more calories. Note that if you exercise a lot more by time and/or intensity, you can take in more calories and still lose weight.

Notice that muscle burns more calories than fat burns. That is not a myth. It is the Truth. Therefore, dieting and aerobics alone are usually not efficient to lose weight. You will need to build muscle. Many women are afraid that if they train, they ill look like a bodybuilder. Do not worry. Unless you train a lot and eat an amount of protein that is a lot more than normal for you, this will not happen. Weight training is good for health, burning calories and your bones.

Weight training also affects insulin resistance due to increased muscle mass. Insulin is a hormone released by the Islets of Langerhans of the pancreas and promotes the uptake of glucose from the blood into cells. Insulin is the body's primary storage hormone because it directs digested nutrients such as glycogen and amino acids into either lean tissue (the liver and muscle) for fuel, or into the fat cells. When you lift weights, your body relies on glycogen for energy. When glycogen fuel stores are depleted, more nutrients are shuttled into muscle cells as opposed to your fat cells. Your metabolism is activated and you burn more calories.

Fat cells are resistant to insulin and glucose. Glucose is more likely to get into muscle cells and get burned. If there are too many fat cells more insulin will be needed. This condition may lead to diabetes. In addition, excess insulin goes to the liver, where it is converted into triglycerides, precursors to fat. Triglycerides interfere with insulin sensitivity, and a vicious cycle ensues.

To find out how many calories you should be burning per day, do an Internet search. It is even better if you consult a physician or dietician. Again, as you work out and get more in touch with your body, you will feel how much food you need per day.

Some information for this section was obtained from the American Cancer Society from internet address http://www.cancer.org/docroot/PED/content/PED_

6_1x_Calorie_Calculator.asp, the Mayo Clinic http://
www.mayoclinic.com/health/metabolism/WT00006/
si=2765 and the Body Muscle Journal http://www.
bodymusclejournal.com/vol03/women_bodyfat_loss.
html.

J. How Many pounds Can You Lose in One Week?

A total of 3,500 calories are in a pound. Carbohydrates
and protein have four calories per gram. Fat has nine
calories per gram.

An intense level of exercise for one hour will be about
600 calories per hour. This varies. A person who runs
very quickly and does interval training will burn more.
This is an average. If one works out at an intermediate
or advanced level at least one hour five days per week,
they can burn at least 500 X 5 = 2,500 calories per
week. If he or she cuts down calories that they eat by
500 calories a week, that is an additional 2,500 calorie
deficit a week. You can also do this by working out
two hours per day for five days at a lower intensity of
250 calories per day. Cardiovascular equipment usually
tells you how many calories you burn after you fill
in statistics like gender and age. You can also consult
textbooks or exercise such as those by the American
Council on Exercise.

Women and men differ by gender, age, health, stress
levels and pregnancy (for women) in how many calories

they burn per week. Usually losing more than three or three and a half pounds per week is not healthy. It may mean a large cut in calories or too much intense exercise, especially if you are a beginner. Also, remember that muscle weighs more than fat. You may want to actually gain weight per week while losing inches in certain areas!

Again, try out your nutrition and exercise plan and see what works and feels good for your soul, mind and body!

K. Log It!

There is nothing like writing it down on paper! For years I have written what I do at the gym on my calendar. According to the period, I have it that I must work out a certain amount of days per month, do certain body parts or exercise a certain amount of time. Writing it down makes it real and helps me to keep track.

Other tricks you may want to try is writing down what you eat each day, morning to night, if you are on a diet. You can keep track of vitamins, nutrients, and calories.

It is also smart to write down your periodic exercise programs. You can do something like this:

Day:	MON	TUE	WED	THR	FRI	SAT	SUN
Muscle Group:							
Abdominal muscles:							
Rectus abdominus							
Obliques							
Transverse obliques							

and so on.

Then you can check which day of the week you worked on what muscle.

Alternatively, you can write the days of the week vertically down the right of the page, and in the squares fill out the exercise or machine, and sets and repetitions for each muscle group and day.

L. Genetics

Everyone is different. For example, two men can work out their biceps doing the same exercise for the same amount of time while on the same diet. One of their biceps may have a different shape or be bigger. If you are working out to look like someone, forget it. You won't. You will only look like you — a variation of you. And that is good news because you are unique and beautiful. And guess what? You were always unique and beautiful even before you starting dieting and working out. Who wants a cookie-cutter body anyway? It's all about taking your body to another level — whether it is a certain muscle, weight, flexibility or strength. It's all a variation of you anyway.

Some people that do aerobics or some female and male bodybuilders, and some female and male strippers look too similar. But they never look alike. Let your body be itself. You may not be able to change some things like proportions or having some cellulite. Embrace it: It is you, it is unique and it is lovely!

Genetics influences how your skeleton is which has a lot to do with posture and length of muscles. It influences from where we tend to lose weight from first. For instance, some women will lose fat from their face that they don't want to lose before they lose all the fat they want to lose from a certain body area. Or they may lose breast fat that they don't want to lose before they lose the abdominal fat that they find it difficult to lose. Remember, you cannot spot reduce. But you can work out and keep in touch with your body to the point that you may be able to influence what you lose from where — much like you can think yourself through an illness and through the pain in a marathon. This cannot be explained so much in words as it can be felt and learned spiritually and through experience.

No matter what, love yourself!

M. Target Heart Rate, Aerobics and Cardiovascular Exercise

You may think that having your heart rate climb to levels when you can feel your heart about to jump out of your chest, or where you are seating profusely means that you are burning fat. That is not necessarily the case. According to the American Council on Exercise, body fat is burned when you exercise at your 60% to 80% heart rate maximum. When you go over this percentage, you are burning glycogen. Aerobics usually has you work at 60% to 80% of your heart rate maximum. That is why aerobics classes, slow jogs and other such exercising can be ideal to burn fat.

At the same time, as was covered before, interval training is key to jolt your body and get you off the plateau. During the fast parts of interval training, you will probably use over 80% of your heart rate maximum. Together with the slow pars, this is a good method to burn fat.

What is your target heart rate? According to the American Heart Association, it is 220 minus your age. For a chart on this, see http://www.americanheart.org/presenter.jhtml?identifier=4736.

Balance and getting to know your body are again key. You will see if you lose more weight by doing more aerobic classes, jogging or weight training at any particular time period. Use time period of three weeks, three months, six months and a year to vary workouts. Of course, if you see that something is not working, you can get off a plateau in between those times.

Weight training is always key because it increases strength and endurance. It also strengthens bones. The increased muscle mass will burn more calories, even when you sit or sleep.

Aerobic training with weight training is key because it is a variation of exercise that will have you use your muscle, endurance and flexibility altogether. Moving around, especially across the floor, is something that incorporates balance and will "shock" the body that has been working out in a stationary fashion with cardiovascular and weight equipment. Interval training may in the end burn more calories because of the "shock" factor in your body. Everyone is different to a degree. You will feel it once you do it and see results in you.

If you use weights four times a week, which is recommended, doing a half-hour aerobics program or jogging from one to four times a week is also recommended. To do this several times a week at a high intensity, you need to be an advanced exerciser. It is a good idea to consult a personal trainer when first beginning to work. You and the personal trainer can monitor your progress and what works best for you. There are people and resources out there that will find you a good aerobics program: books, videos and DVDs, and exercise groups. Abide by the principals of this book of getting to know your body, loving where you are at, and seeing what works for you.

Just as in weight training, it is good to try variety. For instance, try step classes, belly dancing, ballet dancing and different instructors' aerobics programs to see what works best for you. You may want to do two or more different programs in a week. It is best to work out at least 30 minutes in aerobic or cardiovascular activity per day. For the first 20 minutes, your body burns sugar that is readily available in the blood.

The higher your fitness level, the more intensity and time you can put into your aerobic and cardiovascular workouts. If you have been actively enrolled in an aerobics class for six months, you may find that you need to go to a tougher level class or take two classes to get a challenge. You may find yourself almost sleeping through the class while doing what the instructor does. This is an indication that you are on a plateau. Get off quickly! Try a tougher class or at the very least take two classes at this intensity. The first option saves time and gets the same results.

The great thing about cardiovascular machines is that you can vary the intensity. For instance, on a treadmill you can incorporate a slope and on a stair master you can increase resistance. This works your muscles. So you can do an aerobic and muscle strengthening program all in one. This is similar to using heavier weights in parts of an aerobics class where you use free weights or bars.

Once you increase your fitness, your heart will be more efficient. Your stroke volume will increase. That is, your heart muscle will pump out more blood per beat and your heart rate will not increase so easily. You will be able to do more intense exercise while keeping your heart rate at a level where it will burn fat.

Some of the information from this section came from http://www.gurufitness.com/maxfatburn.htm.

Accessed on March 27, 2006

N. Body Mass Index

Knowing your body mass index (BMI) will give you one indication about your health. It has been shown that having a heavier middle or belly is more indicative of a health problem than having heavy hips or legs, especially for women. Your BMI takes this into account. It is calculated by dividing your weight by the square of your height. If you use feet and inches for height, use pounds for weight. If you use meters and centimeters for height, use kilograms for weight. According to the Centers for Disease Control (CDC):

BMI	Weight Status
Below 18.5	Underweight
18.5 – 24.9	Normal
25.0 – 29.9	Overweight
30.0 and Above	Obese

BMI correlates to weight, with differences according to gender and age. Women are more likely to have a larger body fat percentage than men for the same BMI value, and older people are more likely to have more body fat than younger people with the same BMI, according to the CDC.

A high Body Mass Index may be indicative of: cardiovascular disease, high blood pressure, osteoarthritis, diabetes and some cancers, according to Calle EE, et al.

Some information for this section was obtained from http://www.cdc.gov/nccdphp/dnpa/bmi/bmi-adult.htm. and Calle EE, et al. BMI and mortality in prospective cohort of U.S. adults. *New Engl J of Med* 1999;341:1097–1105.

Accessed on March 26, 2006

O. Body Fat Percentage

Body fat percentage depends on your gender and age. Usually, women have a higher body fat percentage than men. It may be acceptable for older people to have a slightly higher fat percentage. Pregnant women definitely for a period of time may have a higher body fat percentage than what is recommended.

This is the body fat percentage chart from the American Council on Exercise:

Classification	Women (% fat)	Men (% fat)
Essential Fat	10-12	2-4
Athletes	14-20	6-13
Fitness	21-24	14-17
Acceptable	25-31	18-25
Obese	32 plus	25 plus

From Health Check Systems
http://www.healthchecksystems.com/bodyfat.htm.

Accessed on March 28, 2006

People often weigh themselves every day. This may help keep you up-to-date on the results of your exercise regimen. However, it may not give you much of a clue. First of all, weight can vary day to day and may be due to things such as a heavy, mostly undigested dinner from the night before, water retention, or the time in the menstrual cycle for women. Perhaps more importantly, after working out for some weeks, you will notice that your muscle mass increases. The same mass of muscle weighs more than the same mass of fat, so you can actually gain weight while you lose a clothing size! Keep these facts in mind when you weigh yourself. It is best to weigh yourself once a week, in the morning after going to the bathroom.

P. Boxing

Boxing is a great cardiovascular work out which also gives you good strength training for the arms and legs, and an incredible mental and spiritual work out. I have done one-on-one training. I cannot begin to imagine what boosts in confidence, security and discipline more training and ring fighting can give.

Boxing is also a great form of interval training. Instructors tell students to do activities such as push-ups, punch the heavy and speed bag, and climb stairs.

Here are some benefits of boxing from the Web site of Steve Franklin http://www.boxingprogram.com/overview.htm.

Benefits from Boxing:

1) The ability to relax, to keep calm and to be poised under pressure

2) A boost in your self-confidence and knowing that you can take care of yourself if necessary in a street fight

3) Faster reflexes

4) Higher strength level

5) Better endurance

6) Quicker movements

7) Improved flexibility

8) Better balance

9) More coordination

Q. Weight

Now we get to an important yet not so important topic: weight. Why is it not so important? It seems like society almost everywhere is getting more and more obsessed with being thin. Thin does not mean healthy. Other factors play into healthy: spirituality, outlook, mentality, genetics, fitness level, strength, flexibility and more. Fat is needed, as shown in a previous section. Having a "high" weight can mean that one has a lot of muscle, which weighs more than fat. Or it can mean that one is tall.

For some people, having a low body fat percentage may be all right, while for other people it is not healthy to have very low body fat and may not even look good.

Regular checkups, balance in diet and endurance, strength and flexibility (which are different for each person), one and, being connected with oneself are all key to fitness. A weight number may be important depending on the individual case, but cannot tell the full story of health, and may mean nothing.

R. Women's Knees

Many athletes and people who work out complain about knee injuries. Knee pain can indicate an injury in a ligament, bursae, or tendon that surrounds the knee joint. It can also indicate arthritis. Women tend to have more cases of certain types of knee injuries than men. One such injury is problems with the anterior cruciate ligament (ACL). This ligament prevents the knee from moving side to side and forward and backward. Some studies have also shown a connection between knee injuries and estrogen. Women are more susceptible to this when their estrogen levels are high, as during ovulation. Women should be extra careful to warm up or stretch leg muscles before and after exercise. Maintaining a healthy weight so as not to place too much stress on the knees is also important. Strengthening leg muscles is key for your fitness.

Several orthopedists have warned women not to wear high-heel shoes. They may have something to do with osteoarthritis, which is seen more often in women over 45 years of age than in men over 45 years of age. High heels may increase rotatory forces in the area where women get osteoarthritis. Osteoarthritis is the most common form of arthritis and affects cartilage, which is the part of joints that cushions them. Osteoarthritis occurs when cartilage gets worn down. If a person has this condition for a long time, their joints can lose their normal shape. Bone spurs can grow at the ends of a joint. Men have more knee cartilage than women, and so are more protected against the condition in their knees than women. In addition, some studies show that elevated estrogen levels exist in women who have osteoarthritis.

S. TV Exercises!

Many times people complain about not having the time to work out. Here you will see that there are no excuses! There are exercises that you can do while watching television! Here are just a few:

1. Get five-pound weights and do some biceps curls, even while sitting on the couch. Sit on the edge of the couch with your back straight and proceed as per the biceps section.

2. Get five-pound weights and do some triceps extension exercises, even while sitting on the couch. Sit on the edge of the couch with your back straight and proceed as per the triceps section.

3. Use free weights for any of the shoulder exercises described in the upper arm and shoulder sections.

4. Use free weights to work out your latissimus dorsi as describe in the latissimus dorsi section.

5. Do jumping jacks! Do four sets of ten repetitions, and walk around for ten seconds in between sets. This basic interval exercise can work out your cardiovascular system quite well!

6. Sit against the wall. That's right, sit against the wall. Keep your knees at a 90-degree angle. This is an isometric squat exercise. It may seem easy, but it may not end up being easy for you! Sit with your back against the wall for ten seconds. Do five sets of ten repetitions. You may break out in a sweat, more than you would when jogging!

7. Jog in place! Do this for a minute at a time. Then walk around for ten seconds. Then do this sequence again two more times. This is a great interval exercise. Use ankle weights or jog for two minutes when you feel that you can.

8. Do the good old abdominal crunch exercise described in the abdominal sections.

9. Sit on the edge of a chair or couch. Keep your back straight. Raise your 90-degree bent legs about three inches from the floor for five seconds. Rest for three seconds. Do this ten times. Does it seem easy? Try it! This works your lower abdominal muscles.

Part III

Some Metabolism and Nutrition Facts

A. Drink Your Water!

It is very important to drink water before, during and after a workout, and throughout the day. About 60% of our body weight is water. Water is key ingredient in many of our body's reactions. Hydrogen and oxygen, which make up water, often dissociate from the water molecule, and go on to be parts of many chemical reactions in our bodies. Hydrogen atoms add to the acidity of molecules, and hydroxide molecules (which are often the result of the disassociation or water), add to the alkalinity of molecules. Thus water contributes to your acid-alkaline balance in your blood and body. Water also aids in digestion.

When you work out and burn calories, you often sweat. This can be a sign that what you are doing is effective. At the same time, it is important to drink water since this will be a key factor in the reactions taking place that your body needs in order to produce energy for your work out. Therefore, water can be a catalyst to weight loss.

It is recommended that you drink at least eight glasses of water per day for good health. As with everything else, get to know your body. Do not drink more water than your body wants per day. This can lead to hyponatremia.

Some information for this section was obtained at the Web site of Joanne Larsen MS, RD LD http://www.dietitian.com/fluids.html., the Department of Molecular Physiology and Biophysics at the University of Vermont http://physioweb.med.uvm.edu/bodyfluids/the.htm. and http://www.freedomfly.net/Articles/Nutrition/nutrition5.htm.

Accessed on November 16, 2005

B. Oxidative Respiration for Muscle Energy

Muscles need energy. This energy comes from food. The food is stored as glycogen in muscles and fat. Sometimes, when there is not much other choice and due to factors such as diet and exercise, the body will burn protein. The fuel for muscle is adenosine triphosphate (ATP). In aerobic respiration, the most common way in which we obtain ATP, the oxygen that we breathe reacts with atoms and molecules to produce ATP. The main fuel for this is glucose, or the most common sugar molecule. Glycogen is reduced to glucose. Here is the reaction:

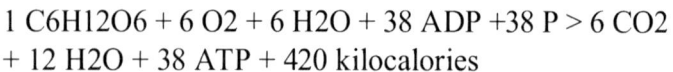

1 C6H12O6 + 6 O2 + 6 H2O + 38 ADP +38 P > 6 CO2 + 12 H2O + 38 ATP + 420 kilocalories

All of the C-H bonds and C-C bonds, which are high in energy, have been lost and replaced by bonds having minimal energy. These minimal energy bonds — H-

O and C-O — have been spared or created. Energy is liberated, along with carbon dioxide, through the oxidation of molecules containing carbon. Note that water is needed for this reaction, so drink plenty of it!

Some information for this section was obtained from http://www.cbu.edu/~seisen/AerobicRespiration.htm.

Accessed on November 22, 2005

C. Lactic Acid - Ouch!

Do you know how your muscles aches after a workout? Sometimes it aches the day after or days later. When oxygen and glycogen in a muscle are used up, the muscle uses anaerobic respiration for energy. As the name infers, oxygen is not used. A product of anaerobic respiration is glucose, which can then be used for aerobic respiration. Pyruvic acid, which is formed from glucose in aerobic respiration, transforms into lactic acid, which diffuses out of the muscle cell into the blood. Energy in the form of adenosine triphosphate (ATP), what muscles use for energy, is produced.

The reaction is:
pyruvate + NADH + H^+ → lactate + NAD^+

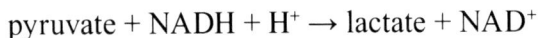

Once sufficient oxygen is restored, the lactic acid can be used for energy or reconverted into glucose by the liver and other tissues (a process known as oxidation).

When too much lactic acid accumulates in the cell, acidity may be too high to maintain the proper degree of acidity in the cell. Fatigue and pain can also result. Resting between sets and resting a muscle used in weight training for at least a day helps to prevent lactic acid-induced fatigue and pain. For some anaerobic sports, such as sprints, it is useful to eat a high glycogen meal after a work out.

Some information for this section was obtained from About Fitness online http://sportsmedicine.about.com/cs/exercisephysiology/a/aa053101a.htm.

Accessed on November 22, 2005

D. Amino Acids

The 20 amino acids of the human body serve as the building blocks of proteins and as the intermediates in metabolism. Proteins not only catalyze most of the reactions in living cells, and control virtually all cellular process. Amino acids determine how a protein will fold into a three-dimensional structure, and the stability of the resulting structure. Meat, especially some meat like chicken and tuna, contains high amounts of protein, as do other foods such as soybeans. That is why bodybuilders often eat huge amounts of these foods — proteins are the primary components of muscle!

Some amino acids are essential; they must be supplied in the food. If a person does not intake even one of the ten essential amino acids, the result can be the degradation of the body's proteins, such as muscle tissue, to obtain the that amino acid. Amino acids are not stored in the human body and the essential amino acids must be in a person's diet every day.

The 10 amino acids that people can produce are alanine, asparagine, aspartic acid, cysteine, glutamic acid, glutamine, glycine, proline, serine and tyrosine. Since tyrosine is produced from phenylalanine, if the diet is deficient in phenylalanine, tyrosine will be required as well. The essential ajmino acids are arginine, histidine, isoleucine, leucine, lysine, methionine, phenylalanine, threonine, tryptophan, and valine.

Diet and exercise go hand in hand. You can consult a physician to find out if you have a deficiency in an amino acid. You can consult a nutritionist for good sources of the essential amino acids.

To see how the amino acids look, check out the Web site of the Institute for Chemistry and Biochemistry at the University of Berlin http://www.chemie.fu-berlin. de/chemistry/bio/amino-acids_en.html.

E. Carbohydrates

Carbohydrates are the most common energy form. They are broken down into sugar, most commonly glucose. They yield four kcal of energy per gram. They come in two basic forms: complex and simple. Simple carbs are a few molecules of sugar linked together in single molecules. Complex carbs are hundreds or even thousands of sugar units linked together in a molecule. Simple sugars are sweet, while complex carbohydrates, such as pasta and potatoes, are pleasant to the taste buds, but not sweet.

There are high-fiber and low-fiber complex carbohydrates. Human beings do not have the enzyme to digest high-fiber carbohydrates like grass. Human beings do not have the enzymes to digest the cellulose in high-fiber, complex carbohydrates. When we eat food with high-fiber, complex carbohydrates, such as certain vegetables, we digest everything but the fiber, which is passed out of our body and actually helps our digestive system do its job. Processing of vegetables strips away fiber and/or vitamin content. One example of processing is cutting an orange and squeezing it for juice, as opposed to just eating it with the white fiber stuck on the flesh of the orange. High-fiber carbohydrates have been associated with lowered incidences of diseases such as hypertension, cancer, arthritis and diabetes.

Some low-fiber, complex carbohydrates are banana, tomato, squash and all cereals and grains, potatoes and rice. The enzyme amylase, which is in human saliva, digests carbohydrates.

When a person eats a simple carbohydrate, the energy is more readily available. However, the person may crash once the energy is depleted. That is why it is recommended to eat a complex carbohydrate such as pasta before a marathon.

If a person eats too many carbohydrates and does not use them as energy, they are converted into fat. As with most other things, a person gets to know their body as they work out, and gets to sense how much of each food group works for their body and for their activity schedule. Of course, getting an annual blood test and physician screening are also important.

F. Protein

Protein comes from Greek πρωτείνη or first thread. Proteins are molecules made up of amino acids. They are complex and have a high molecular weight. Proteins are essential for our body. Some proteins are enzymes or subunits of enzymes. Nutritionally speaking, proteins serve as the source of amino acids. Proteins yield four kilocalories of energy per gram, but they are not the ideal energy source of the body as carbohydrates are.

Adults need a minimum of one gram of protein for every kilogram of body weight per day to keep from slowly breaking down their own tissues for proteins. If a person is malnourished, their body will actually break up muscle cells for protein. Protein malnutrition leads to kwashiorkor. This is most common in children. Symptoms include swollen abdomen, reddish discoloration of the hair and depigmented skin. Protein deficiency can cause growth failure, loss of muscle mass, decreased immunity, weakening of the heart and respiratory system, and death. If someone suffers from kwashiorkor, they are first given food with high content of protein. Digesting protein takes a lot of calcium which comes from food or bone. If you eat too much protein for many weeks, a significant bone mass may occur.

Complete proteins that have all the essential amino acids a person needs come from animals. Vegetarians should eat a variety of protein-containing foods each day and/or should take amino acid supplements.

In the past few years, people have been losing weight using high-protein, low-carbohydrate diets. Some research in the past two years shows that people on those carbohydrate, high-protein diets lose weight quicker than people on low-fat diets. They have shown that after a year or so, weight loss if about equal. This may be so our bodies get on a plateau. These diets may work because: high-protein foods slow the movement of food from the stomach to the intestine, making a person feel full for a longer period of time and feel hungrier later; protein's gentle, steady effect on blood sugar avoids the quick, steep rise in blood sugar and subsequent hunger; and because the body uses more energy to digest protein. You can do your own search on www.pubmed.gov on recent research articles on diets.

Some information for this section was obtained at a Harvard University School of Public Health Web page http://www.hsph.harvard.edu/nutritionsource/protein.html.

Accessed on November 28, 2005

G. Cholesterol and Triglycerides

You must have heard about cholesterol, and how having a high count of this in your section is not good. A high count of the "bad" cholesterol is called hypercholesterolemia and can lead to clogged arteries and heart attack. What is bad cholesterol?

Let's start by a review of what cholesterol is. You can find this information in books and the Internet readily. But this is your quick guide to fitness, so here is a review.

Cholesterol is needed by your body to manufacture some hormones and parts of some cell membranes. Your body makes some cholesterol and ingests other cholesterol from animal products such as meat, poultry, fish, and dairy. Plant food does not have cholesterol. Trans fats and saturated fat causes your body to make more cholesterol.

Low-density lipoprotein, or LDL, is the "bad" cholesterol. LDL can accumulate on artery walls and then lead to atherosclerosis. Too much of it can clog your arteries. The "good" cholesterol is high-density lipoprotein, or HDL. It actually carries cholesterol away from your arteries to your liver where it is eliminated from the body. Some experts believe that HDL removes LDL from artery walls. Some studies suggest that high levels of HDL cholesterol reduce your risk of coronary disease. HDL levels of 35–40 mg/DL are considered normal.

The aim for LDL level should be less than 130 mg/dL for most people. A high LDL level is more than 160 mg/dL, or 130 mg/dL or above if the person has two cardiovascular disease risk factors.

High levels of triglyceride, a form of fat, are not healthy. Triglycerides like cholesterol, are made in the body or ingested. Often people with high levels of LDL have high levels of triglycerides. Triglyceride levels of less than 150 mg/dL are normal. Levels from 150–199 mg/dL are borderline high. Levels of 200–499 mg/dL are high and may indicate the need for treatment in some people.

Ways to increase HDL level and lower LDL level are: eat more monounsaturated and less saturated fat, cut out trans fat, stop smoking, exercise, and eat more fiber. Some physicians recommended drinking one or two alcoholic drinks a day top increase HDL blood level. That seems excessive. But one or two drinks of red wine a week may increase HDL.

Some information from this section was obtained from the American Heart Association

http://www.americanheart.org/presenter.jhtml?identifier=512

H. Moderate Alcohol Intake

My father always told me about Socrates's saying: "Pan metron ariston". That means that everything taken to the extreme is no good. That includes being overly fundamentalist religiously, studying, or working out. This is a central way that I live my life. Perhaps that is why moderate alcohol drinking has been found to be healthy in everything from lowering blood pressure, preventing diabetes, guarding against osteoporosis, keeping away the common cold, and even preventing cancer.

Alcohol molecules end in —OH. Alcohol has been used medicinally throughout recorded history. This use has even been recorded in the Bible. One of the earliest studies that alcohol can be beneficial was in the Journal of the American Medical Association.

Some medical research suggests that alcohol can have a greater impact on heart disease than vigorous exercise, eliminating salt and dieting. I would have to read this research. I am not advocating drinking, but alcohol does dilute the blood, thereby decreasing blood pressure.

Go to www.pubmed.gov and look up "alcohol" or "alcohol and health" to find related scientific journal articles. Do not overdrink. But if you have a glass of wine a day, or I would say every other day or on weekends, you may be furthering your health. This of course depends on where your health is now.

Too much alcohol can be harmful. Pregnant women should not drink alcohol. More on overdrinking will come in a future.

Some information for this section was obtained from http://www2.potsdam.edu/hansondj/ AlcoholAndHealth.html. and a Web page of the State University of New York PotsdamWebMDhttp://www. webmd.com/content/pages/9/1675_57836

Accessed on December 7, 2005

I. Alcohol and the Liver

Alcohol poses damage to the liver when drunk in excess. First, here is a brief overview of the large amount of work that the human liver does: 1. blood detoxification; 2. drug detoxification; 3. glycogen storage; 4. plasma protein synthesis; and 5. production of bile for digestion. Excessive drinking of alcohol can cause alcohol-induced liver disease.

There are three primary types of alcohol-induced liver disease:

1. Fatty liver, which is characterized by the excessive accumulation of fat inside the liver cells. The liver is enlarged and upper abdominal discomfort is often felt on the right side. This is the most common alcohol-induced liver disease.

2. Alcoholic hepatitis is an acute inflammation of the liver, destruction of individual liver cells and scarring. The liver is often enlarged and tender. Symptoms may include fever, jaundice, an increased white blood cell count, and spider-like veins in the skin.

3. Alcoholic cirrhosis is the destruction of normal liver tissue. Non-functioning scar tissue replaces healthy tissue. Symptoms may include those of alcoholic hepatitis, in addition to portal hypertension, enlarged spleen, ascites, kidney failure, and confusion. Alcoholic cirrhosis may lead to liver cancer, which is often fatal. Since the symptoms of alcohol-induced liver disease may resemble symptoms of other medical conditions, consult your physician for a diagnosis.

Some information for this section was obtained from the University of Maryland Medical Center http://www.umm.edu/liver/alcohol.htm.

Accessed on December 8, 2005

Part IV

Stretching

A. Be a Cat with a Friend!

If you have pets, you know how important stretching is to them. My cats, for instance, have relished in their stretches. Have you ever stretched right before getting out of bed and felt like you are giving yourself a long, revitalizing wake-up kiss, like you are in a world of your own?

There are three components of working out. One of them is flexibility. Although this is important, it is often overlooked. Yoga is increasing in popularity and I recommend it. But you can always do a stretch or two on your own while standing or sitting around at home, alone or with a friend. If you use a wall or person for resistance, it can be easier to increase your flexibility. Using a person may be more fun, and they can move you around more than a wall can!

Flexibility increases the range of motion on your joints, which allows you to lift weights and do cardiovascular activity in a more proper way, utilizing more muscle fiber and gaining in strength in a balanced way. Your muscles and spine become supple. Without stretching, you may be more prone to injury and back pain. Studies have shown that stretching may improve circulation to joints and muscle, and may actually help decelerate joint degenerative processes. Stretching is important at the beginning and end of a workout. Stretching warms up your muscles and gets your circulation with important nutrients and electrolytes flowing to the muscle cells. Stretching after a work out can do the same, and can relax the muscles.

Here are examples of stretches to do with a friend:

1. Sit down. Bend forward straight, reaching for your toes. Tell someone to push down on your back in increments of one inch at a time. Tell them to stop if you feel a lot of pain. Hold each position 15 seconds. Breathe. See if each time or day you do this, your hip joint and hamstrings become more flexible. And I am sure this feels good! This is my favorite stretch!

2. Lie down (supine position). Try to keep your lower back flat on the mat or floor. Raise one leg at a time over your head as much as you can. Now, have someone slowly, warning you beforehand, lower your leg millimeters at a time. Tell them to stop if you feel a lot of pain. Hold each position 15 seconds. Breathe. See if each time or day you do this, your hip joint and hamstrings become more flexible. I am sure this feels good!

3. Stretch out one gluteus maximus muscle at a time! Lie down (supine position). Place one leg over your hips, straight out. Bring the toes as high to your waist as you can. Have someone push the leg down and over your hips. Tell them to stop if you feel a lot of pain. Hold each position 15 seconds. Breathe. See if each time or day you do this, your hip joint and hamstrings become more flexible. And I am sure this

feels good! These muscles are the largest and perhaps most powerful of the body! Feel the stretch!

B. Proprioreceptive (PNF) Stretching

Flexibility is an important part of being fit. Stretching is a key way to increase your flexibility. It is important to stretch before and after a workout, especially with the muscles that are in the work out routine. Stretching is a way to warm up and cool down muscles, get blood to your muscle cells, increase the range of motions of joints, and put less stress on joints, muscles and connective tissue.

Proprioreceptors on muscles relay muscle movement information to the central nervous system (CNS). When the muscle stretches to a maximal point, the CNS signals for the muscle to contract. After some seconds, other proprioreceptors signal a relaxation reaction. This all prevents overstraining muscles and injury.

In Proprioreceptive Neuromuscular Facilitation (PNF), the muscle is stretched to a greater degree by increasing the proprioceptor signals through a five – to ten – second voluntary muscle contraction, followed by a five – to ten – second voluntary muscle relaxation. The athlete holds and contracts the muscle against resistance from a partner for ten seconds. The athlete then relaxes, and the partner slowly moves the muscle to a new static position. This is repeated two to three times.

Intermediate and advanced athletes should partake in this type of stretching, and should be overseen by a personal trainer the first time they do it.

Some information from this section was obtained from the Web site of the Hughston Clinic http://www. hughston.com/hha/a.pnf.htm.

Accessed on November 10, 2005

C. Ballistic Stretching and Passive Stretching

Ballistic stretching is really not recommended. It involves the body bobbing up and down forcing a tight stretch out of a muscle. It can be dangerous, leading to pulling a muscle. Ballistic stretching does activate the stretch so the athlete can move with remarkable speed. Ballistic stretching is often done in high school sports. If you are flexible and in intermediate shape, this not a bad idea to do it once in a while to warm up and get the blood flowing. It should not be done more than several seconds at a time.

Passive stretching involves using a partner (or wall) applying additional pressure to increase the intensity of the stretch. Passive stretching is used mainly in gymnastics. It can be dangerous for runners. Passive stretching is sometimes also called relaxed stretching, and as static–passive stretching.

During passive stretching, you assume a position and hold it with some other part of your body, or with the assistance of a partner or some other apparatus. An example is putting your leg on a dancer's bar and bending the other's legs knee, causing the hamstrings to stretch in the leg on the bar. A split is an example of a passive stretch as well. It is good for relieving spasms in muscles that are healing after an injury. It is also very good for "cooling down" after a workout and helps reduce post-workout muscle fatigue, and soreness.

Some of these tips were obtained from the Atlanta Martial Arts Directory http://www.atlantamartialarts. com/articles/stretching/stretching_4.htm#SEC32, a Web page of Lehigh University http://www.lehigh.edu/ dmd1/public/www-data/russ.html. and CM Crossroads http://www.cmcrossroads.com/bradapp/docs/rec/ stretching/stretching_4.html#SEC32

Accessed on November 11, 2005

D. Active Stretching and Dynamic Stretching

Active stretching is also called static–active stretching. In an active stretch, you assume a position and then hold it there with no assistance other than using the strength of your agonist muscles. An example is holding a leg high. It may look easy. People can often kick high. But try holding it for ten seconds! You are stretching your hamstrings. But you need the agonist quadriceps to hold that leg up.

Try it. Even if you have big, strong quadriceps, this may be difficult if you are not used to it.

Active flexibility increases. Agonistic muscles strengthen. These stretches are usually held from between ten and 15 seconds. Many of these are found in various forms of yoga.

When you increase reach, speed or both, you are involved in dynamic stretching. Dynamic stretching, as opposed to ballistic stretching, consists of controlled leg and arm swings that take you to the limits of your range of motion with ease. Ballistic stretches often use force to go beyond a muscle's range of motion. Dynamic stretching is smooth with no bounces or jerks. An example of dynamic stretching would be slow, controlled arm swings or torso twists. Dynamic stretching is good for warm-ups. Sets of about ten repetitions can be performed.

Some information from this section was obtained from

http://www.cmcrossroads.com/bradapp/docs/rec/stretching/stretching_4.html.

Accessed on November 14, 2005

E. Static Stretching and Isometric Stretching

Static stretching is different from passive stretching. Static stretching consists of stretching a muscle or group of muscles to its farthest point and then maintaining or holding that position. Passive stretching consists of a relaxed person who is relaxed while some external force such as a person, apparatus, wall or other, brings the joint through its range of motion.

Isometric stretching is a type of static stretching which involves the resistance of muscle groups through isometric contractions or tensing of the stretched muscles. This increases static-passive flexibility and is much more effective than either passive stretching or active stretching alone. It also helps to develop strength in the "tensed" muscles, which in turn helps to develop static-active flexibility, and it seems to decrease the amount of pain usually associated with stretching. Resistance can be applied manually to one's own limbs, a partner can apply the resistance, or an apparatus such as a wall or the floor can provide resistance.

Examples of manual resistance are holding onto the toes of your foot to keep it from flexing, or putting your leg high on the wall and pressing against the wall, making sure you do not lower your leg. Or a partner could hold your leg up high.

Isometric stretching is an intermediate to advanced movement, and is not recommended for children and adolescents whose bones are still growing, or for people with high blood pressure and osteoporosis. Another type of stretch or warm-up should be done before isometric stretching. Isometric stretching can look easy, but can be straining and can have your hear rate go up. Do this type of stretching if you have been cleared by a physician and are fit. Also, do not do isometric stretches every day. They are to be done a few times a week, month or year, depending on your fitness level and goals. If you do these stretches one day, wait at least two days before you do them again.

To perform an isometric stretch, assume the position of a passive stretch for the desired muscle. The stretched muscle should be stretched for 7-15 seconds. Then, relax the muscle for at least 20 seconds.

When you stretch, some muscle fibers are resting. During an isometric contraction, some of these resting fibers are being pulled upon from both ends by the muscles that are contracting, and they stretch! If you are only performing an isometric stretch, not many muscle fibers contract. But if you are already stretching a muscle, the initial passive stretch overcomes the stretch reflex if you hold the stretch long enough. When you subject it to an isometric contraction, some resting fibers contract and some resting fibers would stretch. Many of the fibers already stretching may be prevented from contracting by the inverse myotatic reflex (the lengthening reaction), and will stretch even more. When the isometric contraction is completed, the contracting fibers return to their resting length, but the stretched fibers will remember their stretched length and will retain the ability to elongate past their previous limit for a period of time. The muscle spindles habituate to an even further-lengthened position.

Some medical studies show that a certain type of stretching for certain periods of time does not always make a difference in health, flexibility, prevention of injury and circulation. Everyone's body is different. Try out warm-up and cool-down stretches for yourself. Getting to know your body is key. See the difference each type of stretch makes at different part of your work out. And vary your stretches throughout the year according to how you feel and results. For medical journal articles, see www.pubmed.gov, which gives free access to Medline, one of the largest databases of medical journals in the world!

Some information for this section was obtained from CM Crossroads http://www.cmcrossroads.com/ bradapp/docs/rec/stretching/stretching_4.html.

Accessed on November 14, 2005

Part V

Muscle Group Exercise Programs

For all exercise programs, drink your water before, during and after exercising to match your body's needs.

Are Skeletal Muscles White or Red?

There are three kinds of muscle: cardiac, visceral (involuntary) and skeletal (voluntary). Skeletal muscles that you use to lift weights in the gym are made up of white and red muscle fiber. How much of each type of muscle fiber we have is genetic.

Thus red muscle tissue contains an extra chemical a special protein-type molecule for oxygen storage called myoglobin. This molecule gives the muscles their red color. The presence of myoglobin in posture muscles enables the sustained contractions for maintaining proper posture and walk. Muscles that depend predominantly on oxidative phosphorylation for ATP require abundant oxygen. Oxygen in these muscles is stored as oxymyoglobin. These muscles are glycolytic, lack appreciable myoglobin and appear white. These muscles generally generate most of their ATP from glycolytic reactions. White muscle fibers generate ATP by a short reaction pathway between substrates such as glucose and the appearance of ATP, whereas in red muscle the pathway from substrate such as glucose to ATP is comprised of many more reaction steps and and is a longer process.

Fast-acting skeletal muscles such as those used by power lifters are composed of dominantly glycolytic white fibers while slow-acting muscles such as those that maintain tone or that are used for marathon running are generally red and oxidative. Most of us have an intermediate balance of white and red muscle fibers. Other people like those that are top marathon runner or power lifters have a predominance of one type of muscle fiber. Most likely, an avid marathon runner could not power lift and an avid power lifter could not run a marathon!

Some Neck Exercises

Usually men do neck exercises to get that bodybuilder look. Most women do not want necks like tree trunks (exaggeration). That is why men train their necks more than women do. However, training your neck once in a while may be good for your neck muscles and posture. After all, your head is heavy and your neck supports your head. Before you embark on a neck exercise routine, consult a physician and a chiropractor. Do all neck exercises slowly and stop if you sense dizziness or pain. Then consult a physician or chiropractor. Do Exercise Routine I or Exercise Routine II once a week.

Exercise Routine I

These are the basic neck movements: neck flexion, neck extension, rotation, side flexion and retraction. Do not use jerky motions. Neck flexion is the movement of bringing the head forward so that the chin hits the chest. Do four sets of ten repetitions. Neck extension is the movement of allowing the head to go back until the face is looking directly at the ceiling. Do this very slowly. Do four sets of ten repetitions. Rotation is turning your head slowly to one side until it cannot easily go any further. Then you turn back the other way. Do four sets of ten repetitions. Do side flexions by keeping your head facing forward and tipping your ear down towards the same shoulder. Do four sets of ten repetitions for each side. Do retraction by keeping your face straight ahead during the whole movement, drawing the head back and the chin down slightly. This neck movement counteracts the tendency of allowing your head to poke forward in a poor posture.

Exercise Routine II

Lie down on a straight bench with your tummy to the bench. Have your collarbone or shoulders by the edge of the bench. Place your hands behind your head. Flex your neck downward. Come back up to starting position. Exhale when you flex your neck and inhale when you move back to the starting position. Do four sets of ten repetitions. For added resistance, you can push against the motion of coming back up to starting position with your hands. Do this after you have done the exercise for three months without resistance if you are a beginner in this exercise.

Lie down on a straight bench with your back against the bench and your shoulders along the edge of the bench.

Extend your neck backward and then go back up to starting position. Inhale when you extend your neck and inhale when you move back to the starting position. Do four sets of ten repetitions. For added resistance, use a circle weight. Use a weight that gives resistance but not pain. Do this after you have done the exercise for three months without resistance if you are a beginner in this exercise.

Sit on the edge of a straight bench. Put on a neck harness. Find a stable position with your back slightly leaning forward at about 45 degrees. Keep your back steady. Flex your neck downward and then back up to starting position. Exhale when you flex your neck and inhale when you move back to the starting position. Use a weight that gives resistance but not pain. Consult a physician and chiropractor before doing this exercise. Do this exercise if you have done neck exercises at least once a week for at least three months before or if you are an intermediate exerciser and feel that you can do it.

Some information for this section was obtained from http://www.bodybuilding.com/fun/exercises. php?MainMuscle=Neck and http://www.bodybuilding. com/fun/exercises.php?MainMuscle=Neck

Accessed on January 5, 2006

Abdominal Muscles

There are four types of abdominal muscles: rectus abdominus, internal obliques, external obliques and transverse abdominus. Different exercises work each of these muscles. People often think they can spot reduce. You cannot spot reduce; genetics play a function in how your muscle will look. Many people with developed abdominal muscles have a rounded look. Two men, for instance, can train their abdominal muscles or biceps with the same exercises during the same time period, and eat the same diet, and end up with muscles that are different sized and shapes. Genetics, including body structure, play a role in this.

One exercise for the rectus abdominus is abdominal crunches. You do not need to come all the way up for this to be effective. You lie on your stomach, place your hands behind your head and come up at a good range of muscle. You can feel when your abdominal muscles are principally working. Use this range of motion. Keep your elbows open. If you keep them closed, your arms are working rather than your abdominal muscles and you can strain your neck. Work in sets and do as many repetitions are a challenge for you without hurting you. A beginner can start with five sets of ten repetitions.

For the internal and external obliques, one exercise you can do to train your transverse obliques is use a broom or weight bar. Hold it behind your neck. Keep your legs open an inch over shoulder width, with knees slightly bent. Keep your back straight. Turn right to left slowly, without bouncing. Work in sets and do as many repetitions as are a challenge for you without hurting yourself. A beginner can start with five sets of ten repetitions.

Transverse obliques are more difficult and subtle to train. We use them when we breathe. One thing you can do to train your transverse obliques is lie down on a small medicine ball. Place the medicine ball beneath your body, right under your septum. Breathe in and out against the medicine ball. Work in sets and do as many repetitions are a challenge for you without hurting you. A beginner can start with five sets of ten repetitions.

Some Swiss Ball Abdominal Exercises

Swiss balls can be great to use because one often needs to incorporate many muscle fibers and muscles to keep one's stability and balance during performance.

Here are some abdominal exercises one can do with a Swiss ball:

1. Get a medium-sized Swiss ball and balance yourself so as to "lie down" on it with your lower back as a pivot point. Place your feet on the ground, with your knees bent 90 degrees. Proceed with abdominal crunches, as described in the first abdominal exercise section. Do five sets of ten repetitions.

2. "Lie down" sideways on the Swiss ball. One leg will be in front of the other on the ground for balance.

Put your hands behind your head. Do side abdominal crunches for your obliques. Exhale when you move upward. Do five sets of ten repetitions one each side.

3. Lie down on the ground. Put the Swiss ball between your ankles. Keep your palms facing downward on your side. Use your lower abdominal muscles. This is a subtle and effective exercise. Bring your hips off the floor about two inches. When you lower your hips, do not have them fully touch the floor. Keep them off the floor for about an inch. When you lift your hips, lift them up to about two inches from this position. You want to target your lower abdominal muscles. Do not use your legs or back to lift the Swiss ball. Do ten sets of ten repetitions. After every five sets, stretch your lower abdominal muscles by hugging your knees for ten seconds.

Three Simple Biceps Exercises

When you work out a muscle or muscle group, you want to target as many muscle fibers as you can, in as many different angles or ways that you can. The biceps are a basic muscle group, composed of two muscles from the shoulder to the elbow. The primarily help you to pull things toward you and to lift things.

It is recommended that you use free weights instead of machines. You have to do more work with free weights, thereby working more muscle fibers and building core balance and strength as well.

Here are three variations of biceps curls with free weights. Choose a weight that gives you a workout, but does not give you severe pain. Choose a weight that you can lift for the full range of motion.

Stand with legs shoulder width apart. Bend your knees slightly. Do not lock your elbows during the exercises. Breathe in when you extend your arm and breathe out when you lift the weight.

1. Lift the free weights from your arms being almost straight smoothly until the free weights almost touch your upper arms. Do four sets of ten repetitions.

2. Repeat [1.] but have your arms point diagonally — 45 degrees from the front of your body.

3. Repeat [2.] and have your inner wrists facing the side of your body.

These variations will allow you to target different muscle fibers and get off a plateau.

Rest in between days where you use the biceps as primary muscles in an exercise. Have fun!

Three Simple Triceps Exercises

When you work out a muscle or muscle group, you want to target as many muscle fibers as you can, in as many different angles or ways that you can. The triceps are a basic muscle group, composed of three muscles from the shoulder to the elbow. They primarily help you to push things away from you or to push your body from a resistance such as a wall or floor.

It is recommended that you use free weights instead of machines. You have to do more work with free weights, thereby working more muscle fibers and building core balance and strength as well.

Choose a weight that gives you a workout, but does not give you severe pain. Choose a weight that you can lift for the full range of motion. Stand with legs shoulder width apart. Bend your knees slightly. Do not lock your elbows during the exercises. Breathe in when you extend your arm and breathe out when you lift the weight.

Here are the exercises:

1. Use free weights that work for you. Hold one arm over your head with a free weight and the elbows bent. Proceed to extend that arm over your head, using the other arm for slight support if you need it. Do four sets of ten repetitions.

2. Bend forward slightly and use one arm to support your weight against a surface such as a weight rack. Hold a free weight with the other arm lifted behind you so that the shoulder and elbow can be as close to 180 degrees as possible. Extend the arm out. Do four sets of ten repetitions.

3. With your arms behind you, hold onto a chair that is secure on the floor. Your legs will be bent or extended before you. Keep your shoulders as low as possible to resting position (not slouching). Use your arms to lift your body up and down. Do four sets of ten repetitions.

As with other muscle groups, rest in between days where you use the triceps as primary muscles in an exercise. Have fun!

Forearms

The forearms are composed of several flexion and extension muscles. For a quick anatomy of forearms, go to www.wikipedia.org and look up "forearms".

Here are simple exercises for wrist flexion and extension.

Wrist flexion - use a barbell:

Preparation:
    It is best to sit. Keep your body stable. Rest your elbows on your thighs. Grasp the bar with an

underhand grip. Let the barbell roll out of the palms down to the fingers. Grip the barbell back up and flex your wrists. Lower steadily and repeat. Do four sets of ten repetitions.

Reverse wrist curl - use a barbell:

Preparation:
Use the same arm and body position. Grasp bar with narrow to shoulder width overhand grip. Rest your forearms on thighs with wrists just beyond knees. Hyperextend your wrist and return until wrist are fully flexed. Repeat for four sets of ten repetitions.

You can incorporate forearm exercises into your exercise routine once or twice a week, depending on how much you want to build them up. Many bodybuilders, especially men, work out the forearms an average of four times a week. Remember to rest them the day after you work them out.

The forearm information from this section was obtained from http://www.exrx.net/WeightExercises/ WristFlexors/BBWristCurl.html.

Rotator Cuff

The rotator cuff is a group of four muscles that helps to lift your shoulders over your head and rotate it toward and away from your body. The muscles are the infraspinaturs, supraspinatus, subscapularis and teres major. Baseball pitchers use these muscles a lot. They are frequently injured by tears, tendonitis, impingement, bursitis and strains.

Shoulder bursitis and rotator cuff tendonitis refer to an inflammation of a particular area within the shoulder joint that is causing a common set of symptoms. They can also be called "impingement syndrome", which indicates an inflammation of the rotator cuff tendons and the bursa that surrounds these tendons. Several bones, muscles, and ligaments contribute to the complex shoulder joint. This increases the chances of injury.

Impingement syndrome occurs when there is inflammation between the top of the humerus or arm bone and the acromion or tip of the shoulder. The tendons of the rotator cuff lie between these bones. In healthy situations, these tendons slide effortlessly within this space. Due to genetics or other factors, the space can become too narrow for normal motion, and the bursa and tendons become inflamed. They thicken and contribute further to the narrowness of the space. The bones rub against each other.

Rotator cuff muscle exercises are often overlooked. A common exercise is often done in grammar school gym classes: arm circles. Have your legs shoulder-width apart and your knees slightly bent. You can do these in the air or against a wall. You can do four sets often small or large circles, in each direction, with each arm. If you do small circles one week, do big circles another week. Do the circles slowly, with a steady posture. Do four sets of ten repetitions with each arm in each direction (moving frontward and backward).

You can also use a rotator cuff machine at the gym. Ask a personal trainer where it is. Have your legs shoulder-width apart and your knees slightly bent. Make sure that your arms, shoulder and back are steady. Just concentrate on moving your rotator cuff muscles. Do four sets often repetitions.

You probably need to work out rotator cuff muscles once every two weeks. Too much working out of these muscles can lead to injury.

You can see four more rotator cuff exercises at http://www.aafp.org/afp/20030315/1315ph.html.

Some information for this section was obtained from the American Academy of Family Physicians http://www.aafp/prg/afp/20030315/1315ph.html. and http://www.jointhealing.com/pages/shoulder/rotator cuff.html.

Accessed on December 29, 2005

Two Simple Latissimus Dorsi Exercises

The latissimus dorsi is one of the largest muscles of the body, and is the largest muscles of the back. It helps define your back and waist. It assists in your bringing objects down from over your heads toward your body or, if you are bent, lifting them from close to the ground to close to your body.

Choose a weight that gives you a workout, but does not give you severe pain. Choose a weight that you can lift for the full range of motion. Do not lock your elbows during the exercises. Breathe in when you extend your arm and breathe out when you lift the weight.

Here are the exercises:

1. Use a pulldown machine. Keep your shoulders relaxed. Grasp the bar and bring it down until the back of your hands barely touch the top of your chest. As you bring the bar down, your shoulder blades will naturally come closer together. Then let it go slowly. Do four sets of ten repetitions.

2. Use free weights. Stand with legs shoulder width apart. Bend forward slightly and use one arm to support your weight against a surface such as a weight rack. Hold a free weight with the other arm. Let the arm almost "dangle" straight in front of your body and to the side (diagonally in front). Lift the weight up until your elbow cannot go higher. When you extend your arm back down, do not lock the elbow. Do four sets of ten repetitions.

As with other muscle groups, rest in between days where you use the latissimus dorsi as primary muscles in an exercise. Have fun!

Some Barbell Exercises

Free weights are generally better to do than barbells since they require more strength from primary and secondary muscle groups to stabilize your movements and posture. Barbells are usually better to do than machines for the same reason. Barbells often do not allow for the variety of motion that free weights or different machines allow.

Gyms usually have several bars of different weights such as 8 pounds, 10 pounds, 12 pounds and 16 pounds. You can use these bars for a variety of exercises with your arms, abdominal muscles and legs. Use a bar weight that will work out your muscles, and will not give you pain. Here are some of these exercises:

Here are some exercises that target different muscles and can be done using barbells:

1. Biceps curls: Choose a barbell weight that will give you a challenge but that you can move for ten repetitions with a full range of motion. Stand with your legs shoulder–width apart and your knees slightly bent. Lift the barbell up until it almost touches your chest, and then down so that your elbows are almost straight. Do not lock your elbows. Do four sets of ten repetitions.

2. Chest press: Choose a barbell weight that will give you a challenge, but that you can move for ten repetitions with a full range of motion. Stand with your legs

shoulder–width apart and your knees slightly bent. Raise the barbell to shoulder level. Push the barbell out until your elbows are almost straight, and then bring it back until it almost touches your chest. Do not lock your elbows. Keep your shoulders relaxed. Do four sets of ten repetitions.

3. Leg muscles: Stand with legs shoulder-width apart and your knees slightly bent to the side diagonally. This time point your toes diagonally out, each toward opposite corners of the room if you are facing the wall. Keep your wrists resting on your quadriceps with your palms facing outward, grasping the barbell. Relax your arms. Sit and get up. Make sure that your knees do not extend beyond your toes. This works your legs muscles and gluteus maximus. It works your adductor muscles especially and is a good variation to cable exercises, squats and lunges. Do five sets of ten repetitions.

4. Triceps: Hold the bar over your head. Keep your elbows straight above you without locking them. Your arms are facing forward. Bend your elbows so that the bar is lowered beneath your head. Return to start position. Do four sets of ten repetitions.

5. Shoulders: Keep your legs shoulder-with apart. Bend your knees slightly. Hold the bar with your palms facing you and your hands touching. Bring it under your chin as you exhale and inhale when you extend your arms. Do not bend your elbows. Do five sets of ten repetitions.

6. Abdominal muscles: Do abdominal crunches with the bar on your belly. Do four sets of ten repetitions.

7. Transverse obliques: Hold the bar behind your neck. Keep your legs a little more than shoulder-width apart and bend the knees slightly. Twist side to side slowly. Twist behind on each side beyond 180 degrees without feeling stress on your side. Do four sets of ten repetitions.

8. Either stand up straight or support yourself against a wall with one arm. Lift up one leg at a time, as a sort of leg extension. Hold the bar with one or two arms over your quadriceps muscle. Lift your leg from the floor to a little more than 90 degrees above your waist, or start about one an a half feet from the floor and lift to the start. Do four sets of ten repetitions with each leg.

9. Lean a little forward and place the bar over the back of one leg. Hold the bar with one arm. Repeat [5.], but lift your leg backwards. Do four sets of ten repetitions with each leg.

10. Do leg abductor exercises by holding the bar, using both arms, so that the bar is "inside" the knee of the leg that you will extend outward, and "outside" the ankle of that leg. Do four sets of ten repetitions with each leg.

11. You can try to hold the bar so that you can do adductor exercises, by holding it in a way that will keep it "inside" both your knee and ankle. If you

can do this, do four sets of ten repetitions with each leg.

12. Do squats with both hands holding the bar over your quadriceps. This is like a pliette ballet move. Keep your legs shoulder-width apart. Keep your back straight. Sit down and then come up as in a squat. Do five sets of ten repetitions.

Some of the information for this section was taken from http://www.self.com/http://www.self.com/http://www.self.com/. Accessed in 2005

More Back Exercises

The back is made up of many muscles. In this section, I will not review back muscles. You can look them up in an anatomy textbook or online. Rather, I will give you some more back exercises.

1. Back row: This exercise works all of the major back muscles, including the rhomboids and trapezius muscles. You can use the weight machine. Machines may differ. See the instructions for position and execution. Some machines have a bar you put across your chest to stabilize your body. Press your chest on the bar so that you are perpendicular to the floor and comfortable. Some even have a seatbelt, which is not needed if you keep yourself steady. Use a weight that gives you a challenge but does not give you real pain.

Pull the cable attachment to waist, and do not lock your elbows when you go back to starting position. Exhale when you pull and inhale when you release. Pull your shoulders back and push your chest forward during the contraction. The shoulders are stretched forward when you return. Do four sets of ten repetitions.

2. Back row cardiovascular machine: The position and movement are similar to the above, but legs are often. Exhale when you pull and inhale when you release. Roll your shoulders back and push your chest forward extended before you on a bar of the machine. You do not have a bar to stabilize your chest. Keep your body and legs relaxed and steady, except for your arms that pull and release the cable. Shoulders are stretched forward when you return. Do this exercise for at least 20 minutes. You can get a cardiovascular and resistance exercise out of this. Once you do this exercise once a week for a month, you can move up to 30 minutes. Feel your body and what it is telling you that you can do.

3. Pull down machine: This exercise is a variation to the cable latissimus dorsi pull down exercise described in another section. There are usually two choices of where to grip the machine. Use variation each time you use the machine. Use a weight that gives you a challenge but does not give you real pain. You pull down the bars to the front of your chest without touching your chest and release without locking your elbows. Exhale when you pull and inhale when you release. Do four sets of ten repetitions.

4. Deadlift: This is a barbell exercise. Use a weight that gives you a challenge but does not give you real pain. Face the bar. Place your legs shoulder-width apart. Bend your knees until your thighs are parallel to the floor. Bend at the waist to lift the bar with an overhand wrist grip. Do not let your knees pass your toes when you bend to grasp the barbell. Straighten your legs as the barbell passes your shins and reaches your knees. Then extend your back until you stand straight. Hold the straightened position for three seconds. Return the bar to the floor by returning to the original position, not by arching or hyperextending your back. Exhale when you pull and inhale when you release. Do four sets of ten repetitions.

Rear Deltoids

Your deltoids, or shoulder muscles, are composed of your front, middle and rear deltoids. Developing rear deltoids also helps to deter shoulder and rotator cuff injuries and to do exercises such as the bench press. Developed rear deltoids look beautiful. There are many exercises that you can do for back deltoids. Two exercises will be reviewed here.

Use the chest fly machine on which you can work out your chest. Adjust the machine arms so that they are at their widest position. This time, sit "backwards" on the machine, with your chest facing the pad. Find a weight that gives you a challenge but does not hurt you. Grasp the handles with your wrists facing you. Relax your back and keep it straight. The full range of motion is pulling the handles backwards. Imagine your shoulder blades moving closer together. Breathe in when you move your arms together. Breathe out when you move your arms apart. Do four sets of ten repetitions.

Use the incline bench. Move it to a 45-degree position. Get barbells where you can repeat the motion that you used in the butterfly machine above. Put your chest against the pad. Raise your arms to shoulder width. Bring your hands together, not touching, with your wrist facing each other. Now extend your arms outward until you cannot extend anymore, without hurting your back. Breathe in when you move your arms inward. Relax your back and keep it straight. Imagine your shoulder blades moving closer together. Breathe in when you return to the start position. Do four sets of ten repetitions.

Some information for this section was obtained from the Web site of Dolfzine Fitness. http://www.dolfzine. com/page526.htm. Accessed on January 4, 2006

Calf Muscles

Human calves are made up of the gastrocnemius muscle and the soleus muscle. The gastrocnemius is the calf muscle that is visible from the outside of the body— it's what makes women's legs look great in high heels and what body builders love to pump. This muscle originates behind the knee on the femur. The Achilles tendon attaches it to the heel. The gastrocnemius is made up of the medial head and the lateral head. This muscle elevates the heel as in plantar flexion. Standing calf raises work the gastrocnemius. Be careful not to hurt your shoulders on the machine. You can actually do this exercise on any raised surface, such as with books, and holds weights for more resistance. This does not strain your shoulders. Do five sets of ten repetitions with a weight that gives you a good work out but does not hurt or strain your muscle.

The soleus is under the gastrocnemius on the rear of the lower leg, and is most active when doing calf exercises where the knee is bent, such as seated calf raises. This muscle also raises the heel, but when the knee is bent. Do five sets of ten repetitions with a weight that gives you a good work out but does not hurt or strain your muscle.

Some information from this section was obtained from http://www.fitstep.com/Advanced/Anatomy/Calves. htm.

Accessed on November 28, 2005

A Week's Quadriceps Training

The quadriceps, or front thigh, muscle group is among the largest in our bodies. Its component muscles are the rectus femoris, the vastus lateralis (externus), the vastus intermedius and the vastus medialis (internus). They are responsible for knee extension (as when you extend your shin forward from your knee) and hip flexion (as when you lie down and extend your legs outward, then bend inward).

When you walk or run, you automatically work your quadriceps. But how many of us, in this day of automobiles, elevators and more do that? All cardiovascular equipment that involves the legs involves the quadriceps. The quadriceps is a large muscle group. The gluteus maximus is the only muscle larger than it is. However, as with all muscles, you want to strengthen your quadriceps for strength and for circulation and bone health. The fact that the quadriceps is so large is optimal for strengthening them to increase your metabolism. As you may already know, this muscle build up will use more oxygen and more energy, and so burn more calories, even when you sit or sleep. Strong quadriceps also improves stability and posture.

This quadriceps section is for intermediate fitness people. Do not forget to first consult a physician before working out and a personal trainer before taking on a new routine.

It is important to rest between quadriceps workouts, so this routine is to be done every other day. It does not include cardiovascular workouts. Do a ten-minute cardiovascular warm up before your quadriceps weights. Afterwards, do a ten-minute cardiovascular cool down. Stretch before your quadriceps workout. One way to stretch your quadriceps is to stand up and hold one leg at a time for at least five seconds bent behind your hips. Do this before and after your weight workout.

Day One:

Do five sets of ten repetitions of leg extension. Use a weight that gives you a workout but not severe pain.

Day Two:

Do four sets of 15 squats. Make sure your legs are shoulder-width apart, you do not lock your knees and you move slowly for the full range of motion.

Day Three:

Do four sets of ten lunges holding a free weight in each hand. Use a weight that gives you a good resistance but not severe pain. One repetition is comprised of both knees going to the floor, in other words, two moves.

Day Four:

Use the lying down leg press machine. Do four sets of ten repetitions with your heels on the edges of the machine. Get up and stretch.

Day Five:

Use a big workout band. They sell them at some gyms and sports good places. Or you can buy them online. Stand. Place one end of the workout band under the ball of a foot. Put the other end of the workout band beneath your other foot. Secure your body against a wall for balance if you need to with the arm opposite the foot with the workout band around it. Lift your foot against the workout band pressure for four sets of ten repetitions. Repeat with the other foot by first changing the workout band positions. What a great workout this is! You will sweat and hardly move!

You may notice that you cannot take a day off in between workouts with these five exercises. So choose three per week and then stick with which three work for you per one-month cycle. Use the same exercises for one month, then change two exercises to get off a plateau!

Four Hamstrings Exercises

The hamstrings are the muscles in the back of the leg: the biceps femoris (long head), biceps femoris (short head), semitendinosus, and semimembranosus. They are responsible for: knee flexion, internal rotation and external rotation and hip extension.

When you work out a muscle or muscle group, you want to target as many muscle fibers as you can, in as many different angles or ways that you can. Choose a weight that gives you a workout, but does not give you severe pain. Choose a weight that you can lift for the full range of motion. Breathe in when you extend your arm and breathe out when you lift the weight.

Here are the exercises:

1. Use the hamstring curl machine. Adjust the seat also that your knees are aligned with the mark, usually a plastic circle on the machine. Hold your back steady.

Use a seat belt if you must. Leave only a little space between the small of your back and the back of the seat. Do smooth, easy movements up and down. Do four sets of ten repetitions.

2. Use the lie-down hamstring curl machine. Make sure that your ankles are beneath the bottom bar that you lift. Do smooth, easy movements up and down. Do four sets of ten repetitions.

3. Lunges (See the "Lunges" section.)

4. Squats (See the "Squats" section.)

As with other muscle groups, rest in between days where you use the hamstrings as primary muscles in an exercise. Have fun!

Cable Leg Adductor and Abductor Exercises

The adductors are a group of muscles that include: the adductor magnus, longus and brevis, the gracilis and the pectineus. They originate on the pelvic bone and attach at intervals along the length of the femur. This interval attachment provides the most power and stability for the hip joint and the femur.

The primary function of the adductors is adduction of the legs, or movement of the legs toward the center line of the body. The adductors also stabilize the hip.

The abductor muscles, on the other hand, abduct the leg away from the centerline of the body. They include the gamelli muscles, piriformis muscle and gluteus minimus.

Do you remember the leg scissor exercises from grammar school? Those worked the adductor and abductor muscles. You can use bands of these muscle groups as well. I will describe a cable exercise to do.

You need to be in shape to do this exercise with a significant amount of weight. Have a personal trainer supervise you for the first time. Choose a weight that gives you a workout, but does not give you severe pain. Choose a weight that you can lift for the full range of motion. Breathe in when you extend your arm and breathe out when you lift the weight.

For the adductor muscles, go to the cable rack. Attach an anklet (most gyms have this) to your right ankle. Move your left leg behind you, to make room for you to steadily move your right leg in front of your left leg and then back like a pendulum. Make sure the weights do not hit. Repeat for four sets of ten repetitions. Repeat for the left leg.

Now put the anklet around your right ankle again. This time face the other way. This will allow you to swing your right leg away from the center line of the body, working the right leg's abductor muscles. Move your leg for the full range of motion. Make sure the weights do not hit each other. Repeat for four sets of ten repetitions. Repeat for the left leg.

As with other muscle groups, rest in between days where you use the adductor and abductor muscles as primary muscles in an exercise. Have fun!

Some of the information for this section was taken from personal trainer Nick Nilsson's Web site Better U Inc. http://www.fitstep.com/Advanced/Anatomy/Adductors. htm.

Accessed on December 20, 2005

Squats

Squats is a powerful exercise that works your lower body — gluteus maximus, quadriceps, and hamstrings as primary movers, and your abdomen, back, and leg adductors and abductors as secondary movers. It is an exercise that strengthens quickly. Women do not have to worry about being too bulky—that comes only with a lot of exercise over time, and with eating an extra amount of protein, over the extra amount of protein you eat because you exercise.

Some fitness professionals and exercisers say that squats are bad for the back and knees. I have experienced back and knee discomfort with squats. Other professionals, as Dr. Fred Hatfield, who is an executive at the International Sports Science Association, has written over 60 exercise books and holds the world record in powerlifting (1,014 pounds) say that squats, if done properly, are not bad of the back and knees. See http://www.drsquat.com/ and www.dolfzine.com/page253.htm. It is best to have the approval or a physician before beginning a squat routine.

Beginners should use an assistant squat rack machine, where the barbell is not free. You may want to start the first three or four weeks with no weight or just a small weight like five pounds on each side of the barbell to practice correct posture. Pick a weight that gives you a workout but not pain. Relax your back and keep your back straight. Keep your legs shoulder width apart. Toes should point just slightly sideways. Place the barbell behind your head. You may find it more comfortable to use a barbell pad provided by most gyms. Grasp the bar strongly with your wrists facing forward. Unhook the bar from the machine. Pretend that you are about to sit down. Sit as deeply as you can. For most people, their thighs will not be parallel with the floor. Each time you do the exercise, you may get closer to this. Make sure that your knees do not move beyond your toes. Inhale when you move downward and exhale when you move back up to the starting position. Move slowly each way. Do four sets of ten repetitions once week.

For squats without a machine, precede the same. Just be careful since it is more difficult. Beginners should use a machine unless they do a light weight. Have someone spot you if you are working at a high weight.

This exercise can also be performed with free weights. Using a bar may be hurtful to your shoulders. If you have major pain, consult a physician. Using free weights is great. Often you cannot use heavy free weights, however, because it proves hurtful to the shoulders.

Again, if you have major pain, consult a physician. To see a squat movement with free weights, see http://www.healthatoz.com/healthatoz/Atoz/hl/fit/demo/squat.jsp.

If you are an advanced exerciser, having done squats weekly for at least six months, plyometric squats and lunges work well for leg muscles, including quadriceps. Rest your quadriceps for at least a day in between working them out on leg machines or plyometric movements.

Some information for this section was obtained from http://www.exrx.net/ExInfo/Squats.html., http://www.dolfzine.com/page253.htm. and http://www.healthatoz.com/healthatoz/Atoz/hl/fit/demo/squat.jsp.

Accessed January 6, 2006

Lunges

Lunges are an effective leg exercise that work out your quadriceps, hamstrings, gluteus maximus, and, to a lesser extent, your abdominal, adductor and abductor muscles. Your abdominal, back and hip muscles are used as stabilizers.

You can perform lunges in a stationary fashion or while moving across the floor. You can do what feels best or yields the best results. Do lunges once a week. You may want to alternate weeks between stationary and moving lunges. Pick a weight that gives you a workout yet not the bad kind of pain. Keep your back straight and do not bounce.

You can use a free weight in each hand or a barbell across your shoulders. Stand up straight with your feet shoulder width apart and your knees partly bent. Step forward with your right leg. Make a 90–degree angle with your right leg. Your thigh should end up parallel to the floor. Bend your knees until your left knee is only an inch from the ground. Push up and back with your right leg while keeping your back and body steady until you are in the starting position. Repeat with the opposite leg. Do five sets of ten repetitions. Each repetition is composed of one two movements, each movement with an alternate leg stepping forward.

To see an animation of stationary lunges, go to http://www.theministryoffitness.com/mof/library/anims/llunges.htm.

Some information for this section was obtained from http://www.betterbodz.com/quariceps/free weight_lunges.html. and http://www.theministryoffitness.com/mof/library/anims/lunges.htm. Accessed on January 9, 2006

Possible Arm Three-Month Exercise Routine I

Here is a possible three-month program to sculpt your upper arms. Feel your body and look in the mirror to see results. If these exercises do not seem to work, increase the repetitions or sets, or use a substitute exercise. For all of the exercises, exhale when you lift the weight or exert the most muscle tension, and inhale when you return to the beginning position. Use a weight that gives you a workout but is not too tough. Rest the muscle in between days that you work it out as a primary mover.

Biceps curls twice a week:

Day One: Use free weights. Do five sets of ten repetitions.

Day Two: Use a barbell. Do five sets of ten repetitions of biceps curls.

Triceps twice a week:

Day One: Do the overhead triceps exercise one free weight at a time. Do five sets of ten repetitions.

Day Two: Use a cable machine with a small bar. Adjust the weight on the machine. Do five sets of ten repetitions.

Shoulders:

Use the overhead press machine. Do five sets of ten repetitions.

Use free weights. Pick a weight that you are comfortable with and that will give you a good workout. Stand with legs shoulder-width apart and knees bent. Keep your back straight. Grasp the free weights with your palms facing toward you. Lift the free weights with your elbows pointing out, perpendicular to your body. Lift until the weights come under but not touching your chin. Repeat without locking your elbows. Do five sets of ten repetitions.

Look at the rotator cuff section for rotator cuff exercises. Do one exercise a week, alternating between the "circles" exercise and the rotator cuff machine exercise.

Rest each primary muscle group for a day after you exercise it. For instance, do not do a biceps exercise the day after you use your biceps as a primary muscle in an exercise, such as the biceps curl. You may do a shoulder, rotator cuff or forearm exercise (see next session) as well. This week's routine can look like:

Monday	Tuesday	Wednesday	Thursday
Biceps	Triceps	Biceps	Triceps
Shoulders	Rotator Cuff	Shoulders	Forearms

Friday	Saturday	Sunday
Rest arms	Biceps	Rest arms

Possible Arm Three-Month Exercise Routine II

Here is a possible three-month program to sculpt your upper arms. Feel your body and look in the mirror to see results. If these exercises do not seem to work, increase the repetitions or sets, or use a substitute exercise. For all of the exercises, exhale when you lift the weight or exert the most muscle tension, and inhale when you return to the beginning position. Use a weight that gives you a workout but is not too tough. Rest the muscle in between days that you work it out as a primary mover.

Day One:
   Use the Gravitron machine. Ask a personal trainer if you do not know which machine it is. Put the pin at the amount of weight you want the machine to lift. If you subtract this from your body weight, that is the amount of weight that your body is lifting. The machine will have an illustration of the two basic movements — pull ups, that work the biceps and upper back (secondary) muscles, and pull downs or dips, that work the triceps and chest (secondary) muscles.

   Do five sets of ten repetitions of pull ups.
   Do five sets of ten repetitions of pull downs.

Day Two:
   Use a biceps (arm curl) machine. Do five sets of ten repetitions of biceps curls.

Since you are doing biceps once a week, use a weight that challenges you and does not give you pain.

Day Three:

Use a triceps (arm extension) machine. Do five sets of ten repetitions. Since you are doing triceps once a week, use a weight that challenges you and does not give you pain.

Day Four:

Use free weights to work out your shoulders. Pick a weight that you are comfortable with and that will give you a good workout. Stand with legs shoulder-width apart and knees bent. Keep your back straight. Grasp the free weights with your palms facing toward you. Lift the weights with each arm to your side. Lift the weights slowly and then lower the weights slowly. Repeat without locking your elbows. Do five sets of ten repetitions.

Possible Three-Month Arm Exercise Program III

Here is a possible three-month program to sculpt your upper arms. Feel your body and look in the mirror to see results. If these exercises do not seem to work, increase the repetitions or sets, or use a substitute exercise. For all of the exercises, exhale when you lift the weight or exert the most muscle tension, and inhale when you return to the beginning position. Use a weight that gives you a workout but is not too tough. Rest the muscle in between days that you work it out as a primary mover.

Day One:

Biceps:
Use a barbell for biceps curls. Do five sets of ten repetitions.

Day Two:

Triceps:
Use the cable rack. Use the rope attachment. Ask a personal trainer if you do not know which attachment that is. Find the right weight according to the first paragraph's instructions. Do this exercise as you would with a bar, but as you extend your forearms past your elbows, start to slowly separate the two ends of the rope until you do so as much as you can (while not extending your elbows totally). Ask a personal trainer if you cannot figure this out by these instructions.

Day Three:

Shoulders:
Use the overhead press machine. The instructions on the machine are easy to follow. Do five sets of ten repetitions.

Day Four:

Shoulders — Front deltoids:
Pick free weights that will give you a good work out, but not pain. Stand with your legs shoulder-width apart and knees slightly bent. Bring one arm extended (with elbow almost fully extended) in front of you one at a time until your arm is shoulder level. Do four sets of ten repetitions. One repetition will be each arm coming up to shoulder length.

Rear deltoids:
Use the rear deltoid machine. The instructions on the machine are self-explanatory. Use an amount of weight that will give you a good work out, but not pain. One motion is pulling the weights toward you and one is releasing them away from you. Do both movements slowly. Ask a personal trainer or use the instructions on machine. Do four sets of ten repetitions.

Possible Three-Month Chest
Exercise Program I

Here is a possible three-month program for your chest. Ladies, do not worry, you will not lose your breasts and look like a man, although you could if you want. Your chest muscles will tighten up. This will make you be strong and feel great. And you will look great, too. Your breasts will lift, although if you have sagging or huge breasts, they will not look very different. The breasts are made up of adipose (fat) tissue. The pectoralis muscles and intercostal (between the ribs) muscles will be worked out; your breasts will mainly stay the same. To reduce breast size, you do cardiovascular exercises, as well as overall weight training. To not lose breast adipose tissue, which concerns mostly women when they work out, is more difficult. You cannot tell your body what to do. Genetics partly or mostly determines what you lose from where first. You may be working out your legs mostly, but in a period of time lose mostly breast adipose tissue. You can feel your body, and use your spirituality and mentality to affect results. This is something you learn on your own.

Feel your body and look in the mirror to see results. If these exercises do not seem to work, increase the repetitions or sets, or use a substitute exercise. For all of the exercises, exhale when you lift the weight or exert the most muscle tension, and inhale when you return to the beginning position. Use a weight that gives you a workout but is not too tough. Rest the muscle in between days that you work it out as a primary mover.

Day One: Supine Chest Press

Lie down on a flat bench with your free weights, one in each hand. With your feet flat on the end of the bench or on the floor, and make sure there is only a small natural space between the small of your back and the bench. With your wrists facing each other, start by extending your arms to your sides (right arm to right side and left arm to left side). Then bring your wrists together without having the weights touch. Do four sets of ten repetitions. You can repeat another four sets of ten repetitions with your wrists facing forward.

Day Two: Chest Fly Machine

Use a chest fly machine. Adjust the arms of the machine to go as far backward as possible. Make sure that the seat position is comfortable. Bring your arms together. Do four sets of ten repetitions.

Day Three: Bench Press

Use the bench press. Find the weight that is right for you and balance it on each side of the bar. Lie down with your back relaxed, only an inch or two separating your lower back from the bench. Lift the bar in slow, steady movements from about two inches over your chest until your elbows are straight, but not locked. Do four sets of ten repetitions.

Possible Three-Month Chest Exercise Program II

Choose a weight that gives you a workout, but does not give you severe pain. Choose a weight that you can lift for the full range of motion. Breathe in when you extend your arms and breathe out when you lift the weight.

Here are the exercises:

Day One: Supine Chest Bench

Lie down on a flat bench with your free weights, one in each hand. With your feet flat on the end of the bench or on the floor, make sure there is only a small natural space between the small of your back and the bench. With your wrists facing each other, right and left, start by extending your arms to your sides (right arm to right side and left arm to left side). Then bring your wrists together without having the weights touch. Do four sets of ten repetitions. You can repeat another four sets of ten repetitions with your wrists facing forward.

Day Two: Chest Fly Machine

Adjust the arms of the machine to go as far backward as possible. Make sure that the seat position is comfortable. Bring your arms together. Do four sets of ten repetitions.

Day Three: Incline Chest Press Machine

The instructions on the machine are self-explanatory. Do four sets of ten repetitions.

Day Four: Bench Press

Find the weight that is right for you and balance it on each side. Repeat the back position of [1.]. Do four sets of ten repetitions

As with other muscle groups, rest in between days where you use the pectoralis major and minor muscles as the primary muscle groups in an exercise. Pay attention to how your body responds to each exercise. Have fun!

Possible Three-Month Chest Exercise Program III

Here is a possible three-month program for your chest. For all of the exercises, exhale when you lift the weight or exert the most muscle tension, and inhale when you return to the beginning position. Use a weight that gives you a workout but is not too tough. Rest the muscle in between days that you work it out as a primary mover.

Day One: Incline Chest Press

See prior section. Have your wrists face each other as you hold the free weights. Do four sets of ten repetitions. Now repeat while having your wrist facing forward. Do four sets of ten repetitions. Rest two days after Day One.

Day Two: Cable Machine

Stand with legs shoulder width apart. You may find it easier to balance by putting one leg about a foot in front of the other. Bring the cables closer together, and then release them slowly. Exhale when you bring the cables closer, and inhale when you bring the cables further apart. Do not let the weights rest until the end of each set. Perform the exercise slowly. You may want to ask a personal trainer to demonstrate. Do four sets of ten repetitions.

Day Three: Medicine Ball

You will need a partner! This can be fun! Throw the medicine ball in rhythmic slow and powerful motions between yourselves at upper rib level. Do four sets of ten repetitions.

Possible Three-Month Chest Exercise Program IV

Here is a possible three-month program for your chest. For all of the exercises, exhale when you lift the weight or exert the most muscle tension, and inhale when you return to the beginning position. Use a weight that gives you a workout but is not too tough. Rest the muscle in between days that you work it out as a primary mover.

Day One: Push Ups

Put your palms on the floor, shoulder width apart, fingers facing forward. Keep your toes on the floor. Keep your back straight. Extend and bend your elbows in slow, smooth motions. Never fully extend your elbows. Exhale when you move up and inhale when you move down. Do five sets of ten repetitions.

Day Two: Bench Press

See the first chest exercise program section. Do five sets of ten repetitions. Rest your chest for two days after this exercise.

Day Three: Cable Rack:

See the prior section. Do five sets of ten repetitions.

Three-Month Abdominal Exercise Program I

The front abdominal muscles are one straight muscle, the rectus abdominis, and the three flat muscles, external oblique, internal oblique, and transversus abdominis.

There are many ways that you can work out your abdominal muscles. Try this weekly work out for three months. See if you get results in how you feel, abdominal strength and how you look. Then move on to the abdominal program for another three months. As usual, rest your abdominal muscles as primary movers the day after your work them out as primary movers. There is almost no exercise which does not incorporate the abdominal muscles as secondary movers, or stabilizers.

Day One:

Do five sets of ten repetitions of abdominal crunches. This is the correct way to do them.

Lie on the floor with about an inch or two inches of natural space between the small of your back and the floor. Put your hands behind your head. Relax your arms and shoulders. Keep your back straight. Do not curve your neck. Do not use your arms to come up. You only need to lift your upper body about 20 degrees from the floor. You will feel when you have reached your limits. Keep your elbows straight out and perpendicular to the floor. Concentrate on using your abdominal muscles. Exhale when you move up and inhale when you move down. Pretend that there is an imaginary rope from your septum (chest bone) to the ceiling pulling you up in a straight fashion.

Day Two:

Grab a medium-sized Swiss ball. Lie on the floor with about an inch or two inches of natural space between the small of your back and the floor. Put the Swiss ball between your knees. Keep it there with your leg muscles. With the top of your body relaxed and your waist on the floor, lift only your hips about two inches from the floor using your lower abdominal muscles. Inhale when you move your legs up and exhale when you move your legs down. Do five sets of ten repetitions.

Day Three:

This exercise works your oblique muscles. Take a weight bar. If you are a beginner, take a light weight bar, such as a five–pound bar or an eight-pound bar. Place the weight bar behind your neck and hold it with your wrist facing forward. Stand with your legs shoulder-width apart and knees slightly bent. Relax your back and shoulders. Turn slowly right to left with the bar to a comfortable position on each side. Do five sets of ten repetitions.

Three-Month Abdominal Exercise Program II

The front abdominal muscles are one straight muscle, the rectus abdominis) and the three flat muscles, external oblique, internal oblique, and transversus abdominis.

There are many ways that you can work out your abdominal muscles. Try this weekly work out for three months. See if you get results in how you feel, abdominal strength and how you look. Then move on to another abdominal exercise program for another three months. As usual, rest your abdominal muscles as primary movers the day after your work them out as primary movers. There is almost no exercise which does not incorporate the abdominal muscles as secondary movers, or stabilizers.

Day One:

Use the abdominal crunches machine. There is a pad that you place in front of your chest. Sit comfortably and relax your body. There is usually a pad for your head. Let your arms rest loosely next to you. Find a weight that gives you a workout but not unduly pain. Often when you work out your abdominal muscles, you will not feel the pain until a day or two after your workout. Exhale when you move forward and inhale when you move up to the starting position. Do five sets of ten repetitions.

Day Two:

Use the cable rack. Adjust the pulley where the cable attaches to the highest level. Place a handle on the hook that is a loop that both of your hands can hold onto, or a metal attachment that has a place for each of your hands to hold.

Find a weight that gives you a workout but not unduly pain. Hold the attachment and bring it with you to the floor. Sit on your knees. Bring the attachment in front of the top of your chest bone or septum. Keep your neck aligned with your back and your back relaxed and straight. Move all the way up, holding the attachment in the same position. This is the starting position. Move downward so that your hands that are holding on to the attachment almost touch the floor. Exhale as you move downward. Move up to the starting position. Inhale when you move up to the starting position. Do not let the weights touch. Do five sets of ten repetitions.

Day Three:

This exercise works your oblique muscles. Lie on the floor with your knees bent. The natural space between the small of your back and the floor should be about two inches. Relax. Place your hand behind your head. Lift your upper body from the waist up. Concentrate on using your oblique muscles. Have your left breast almost touch your right knee. Slightly move back about an inch and have your right breast almost touch your left knee. Do five sets of ten repetitions.

Three-Month Abdominal Exercise Program III

Here is another abdominal exercise program. Rest the muscle in between days that you work it out as a primary mover. The first day is like the Three-Month Abdominal Exercise Program I first day exercise. You can vary it, perhaps causing different muscle fibers to be used, by holding your legs crossed straight up in they air or against a wall.

Day One:

Do five sets of ten repetitions of abdominal crunches. See the Three-Month Abdominal Exercise Program I.

Day Two:

Lie on the floor, allowing the slope of your back to have a natural curve. There will be a space of about an inch an a half between the small of your back and the floor. Place your arms straight along your sides, or under the outer part of your buttocks, with the palms facing downward for leverage. Or you can hold onto to something like the leg of a bed with one or both arms. Lift your legs straight and close together in front of you slowly up and down. Inhale as you bring your legs up, and exhale as you bring your legs down. Do not fully relax your legs. In other words, do not release the movement until the set is done. Do five sets of ten repetitions. This exercise works your lower abdominal muscles as stabilizers. The heavier, in muscle or fat, your legs are, the more of a workout your lower abdominal muscles will get. If you would like to make this exercise tougher, hold your legs in an isometric movement for three to ten seconds, whatever you can do, about two inches above the ground at the end of this movement. Do this only if you are an intermediate exerciser or have done this exercise for about a month.

Day Three:

Use the abdominal machine where you support yourself on your arms by holding onto handles and placing your forearms on pads. Ask a personal trainer if you cannot find this machine. This exercise works your lower abdominal muscles as stabilizers. Stabilize your upper body. Bring your legs straight up in front of you up to your waist and then bring them slowly back down without fully relaxing your legs. In other words, do not release the movement until the set is done. Exhale as you bring your legs up, and inhale as you bring your legs down. Do five sets of ten repetitions. Now do the same thing, just lift your legs on the right side for five sets of ten repetitions. This works your right oblique muscles. Then lift your legs on the left side for five sets of ten repetitions. This works your left oblique muscles. The breathing is the same: exhale when you bring your legs up and inhale when you bring your legs down. These above exercises can be done with bent knees. Use whatever leg position that brings you the results that you want. It tends to be tougher with straight leg. If you are a beginner, you may want to start with a bent knee.

Three-Month Abdominal Exercise Program IV

These are advanced abdominal exercises to be done after doing each of the prior abdominal exercise programs for at least one month each, or if you are an advanced exerciser, working out your abdominal muscles at least two times a week for two years.

Day One:

Sit on a mat with your left knee bent and left foot flat on the mat. Place your right ankle over your left knee and your hands behind your head. Rest your head on your hands and keep your back straight. Do an abdominal crunch and then more your midline to your right knee, without touching, for a left oblique workout. Repeat this for four sets of ten repetitions. Then do the same while changing position: Bend your right knee with your right foot flat on the mat. Place your left ankle over your right knee. Rest your head on your hands and keep your back straight. Do an abdominal crunch and then more your midline to your right knee, without touching, for a right oblique workout. Repeat this for four sets of ten repetitions.

Day Two:

The "Rotator" - Sit on a mat and bend your knees. Imagine a pole from your belly button to the ceiling. You will rotate about a foot around this pole with your hands behind your head. Rest your head on your hands and keep your back straight. Move from the back position right and forward, left and back to the first position. You can go left for variety. Do this for five sets of ten repetitions.

Day Three:

Use a medicine ball of ten pounds or less —
whatever you can handle and that gives you workout.
Sit on a mat with knees bent. Hold the medicine
ball with your arms straight over your head. Do
regular abdominal crunches while holding your
arms straight above your head as you complete the
move. An easier version is holding the ball with
bent arms under your septum. Do this for five sets
of ten repetitions.

Three-Month Abdominal Exercise Program V

Here is another abdominal exercise program. This is an
advanced program. Do this program after at least one
month each of doing the previous abdominal exercise
programs. Rest the muscle in between days that you
work it out as a primary mover. The first day is like
the Three-Month Abdominal Exercise Program I first
day exercise. You can vary it, perhaps causing different
muscle fibers to be used, by holding your legs crossed
straight up in they air or against a wall.

Day One:

Do five sets of ten repetitions of abdominal crunches.
See the Three-Month Abdominal Exercise Program
I.

Day Two:

Get arm rests (ask a personal trainer) that you can hook onto the top bar of a cable rack, squat rack or other machine. Get a step or two (ask a personal trainer) to get your arms onto the rests. Your elbows should stick out of the arm rests and your hands should clasp the top part of the arm rests. Your forearms should be 90 degrees with the floor. Step off the step(s) and relax your body. Keep your upper body relaxed and straight. Lift your legs upward and then downward. Alternatively, you can bend your knees and bring your upper legs up to your hips. Then in a small motion, bring your legs up one to two inches from your hips. This works your lower abdominal muscles at about the same intensity as the prior motion. See what feels best for you and brings the best results. Exhale when you move your legs up and inhale when you move your legs down for either way of doing the exercise. Do five sets of ten repetitions.

Day Three:

Do the advanced abdominal exercise from the "Perhaps the Best Abdominal Exercise" section.

Possible Three-Month Leg Exercise Program I

There are almost countless exercises that you can do for legs. Here is a possible three-month program to sculpt your legs. Feel your body and look in the mirror to see results. If these exercises do not seem to work, increase the repetitions or sets, or use a substitute exercise. For all of the exercises, exhale when you lift the weight or exert the most muscle tension, and inhale when you return to the beginning position. Use a weight that gives you a workout but is not too tough. Rest the muscle in between days that you work it out as a primary mover. Do a calf exercise at least once a week. See Part II, Section E, "Calf Muscles".

Quadriceps twice a week:

Use the leg extension machine. The exercise is described in the quadriceps section. Do four sets of ten repetitions.

Hamstrings twice a week:

Use the leg curl machine. This exercise was described in the hamstrings section. Do four sets of ten repetitions.

Adductor and Abductor Exercises:

Alternate weekly between using the adductor and abductor machines and the cable exercises.

For the adductor and abductor machines:

These machines have two pads each. Ask a personal trainer if you cannot find them. For the adductor machine, sit with your legs "outside" the pads. Unhook the pads so that they can move. There is a handle for this. The motion is to move your legs closer together and then farther apart. Choose a weight that will give you a good workout and that will not hurt you. Exhale when you move your legs inward. Inhale when you move your legs outward. Be sure not to have the weights touch when you move the legs outward. Do four sets of ten repetitions.

For the abductor machine, sit with your legs "inside" the pads. Again, choose a weight that will give you a good workout and that will not hurt you. Move your legs inward and outward. Again, be sure not to have the weights touch when you move the legs outward. Exhale when you move the pads outward. Inhale when you move the pads inward. Do four sets of ten repetitions.

Overall Legs twice a week:

Use the squat rack once a week. See the squats section. For beginners, use the one that assists you. In other words, the barbell is not loose. Put the bar behind you. Have your legs shoulder-width apart and knees bent. Unhook the barbell. Keep your back straight. Pretend that you are sitting. "Sit" until you are comfortable, making sure that your knees do not go beyond your toes. Stand back up and repeat for four sets of ten repetitions. Notice if you have back or knee pain. This can be a strenuous exercise. Notify a physician if you have pain.

Use the leg press machine once a week. Put your legs about shoulder width apart. Do four sets of ten repetitions, without touching the weights when you go back to beginning position.

Possible Three-Month Leg Exercise Program II

Quadriceps twice a week:

Use the leg extension machine. The exercise is described in the quadriceps section. Do four sets of ten repetitions.

Hamstrings twice a week:

Use the leg curl machine where you lift one leg at a time. You may find that this is harder than using the leg curl machine where you bend both legs at once. (You can also do one leg at a time on this machine.) Adjust the machine so that you use the leg that you want to use and rest the leg that you are not using. You may have to ask a personal trainer to help you the first time. During the workout, only use the leg that you are exercising. Relax the rest of your body. Use slow motion to lift the leg and to lower the leg. This exercise was described in the hamstrings section. Do four sets of ten repetitions.

Adductor and Abductor Exercises:

Alternate weekly between using the adductor and abductor machines and the cable exercises for the same muscles. See the prior section. Do four sets of ten repetitions.

Overall Legs twice a week:

Do lunges. See the "Lunges" section. Do five sets of ten repetitions.

Possible Three-Month Leg Exercise Program III

Lunges twice a week:

See the lunges section for instructions.

Overall legs twice a week:

Use the leg press machine. Use the leg press machine where you have your legs above you once a week. Use the leg press machine where you are horizontal once a week. Do four sets of ten repetitions. For two sets of repetitions, have your legs close together. For two sets of repetitions, have your legs apart, putting your heels on the corner of the leg press machine.

Do four sets of ten repetitions for calves. Put the ball of your feet on the edge of the leg press machine. Move your feet to move the weights up and down.

Gluteus Maximus

The gluteus maximus is the strongest and biggest muscle on the human body. It is responsible for the following hip movements: adduction (moving the thigh inward with hip straight), transverse abduction (abduction of the leg with hip bent as in sitting), extension (moving the thigh or top of pelvis backward), and external rotation (rotating the leg away from the body). This muscle is important for balance, walking, and running.

Squats and leg abductor exercises engage the gluteus maximus muscle. The gym machine the "Butt-Blaster" also works the gluteus maximus primarily. Here is a possible three-month exercise program for the gluteus maximus. You can count your squat days as a gluteus maximus and leg day.

Day One:

Squats (See the "Squats" Section.)

Day Two:

Use the Butt-Blaster machine. The instructions on the machine are self-explanatory. Move slowly and steadily. Do five sets of ten repetitions.

Day Three:

Cable Abductors (see the "Cable Leg Adductor and Abductor Exercises" Section .)

For more gluteus maximus exercises, see http://www. exrx.net/Lists/ExList/HipsWt.htmeu

Some information for this section was obtained from http://www.betterbodz.com/quariceps/free weight_ lunges.html. and http://www.theministryoffitness.com/ mof/library/anims/llunges.htm.

Accessed on January 9, 2006

Gluteus Minimus and Gluteus Medius

The gluteus minimus is a tiny muscle of the hip that is covered by the gluteus maximus. It helps in the following motions: hip abduction (moving the leg away from the body), transverse abduction (abduction of the leg with hip bent as in sitting), and internal rotation (rotating the leg away from the body).

The gluteus medius is also hidden by the gluteus maximus, which is responsible for the same movements and for external rotation (rotating the leg away from the body).

You can work the gluteus minimus and the gluteus maximus with gluteus maximus exercises. (See the "Gluteus Maximus" Section.)

Some information for this section was obtained from http://www.exrx.net/Muscles/GluteusMinimus.html. and http://www.exrx.net/Muscles/GluteusMedius.html. Accessed on January 11, 2006

Conclusion

Read this book more than once. Before training, get a medical checkup and ask the physician if any exercises are contraindicated for you. You may want to consult a personal trainer for ten or more sessions. Try the programs. Read the first part over and really get it. Feel your spirit, intellect, emotions and body through your journey of working out.

The last poem in my book *Life, Work and Play: Poems and Short Stories* is about being true to yourself, reaching your goals, liking how you look and just being you! You can find my books on www.louizapatsis.com, www.authorhouse.com, www.amazon.com, and www.bn.com. Search by my name Louiza Patsis or by title.

About the Author

Louiza Patsis has been working out intermittently since she was nine years old. She first worked out in a gym at her high school St. Francis Prep in Fresh Meadows, NY. She did not begin to work out regularly in a gym doing cardiovascular work and lifting weights until December 2003. Ms. Patsis has run in seven marathons and three half marathons. She has not stopped for over 12 years.

Ms. Patsis also has a Bachelor's of Arts in Chemistry and Masters of Science in Biology from New York University. She is the President of LP Enterprises. Ms. Patsis in the past has been certified as a personal trainer by the American Council on Exercise, the American College of Sports Medicine and the International Sports Sciences Association.

Louiza Patsis is the author of *The Boy in a Wheelchair*, which she wrote at 10 years old. It tells the story of a boy who is physically challenged and bullied, and yet excels in school and plays sports. She is also the author of *Life, Work and Play: Poems and Short Stories*, a collection of works written in the span of 12 years.

To order, call LP Enterprises at (212) 252 – 6947, or send an email to PocketGuidetoFitness@yahoo.com.

Printed in the United States
74150LV00001B/1-99

9 781425 956752